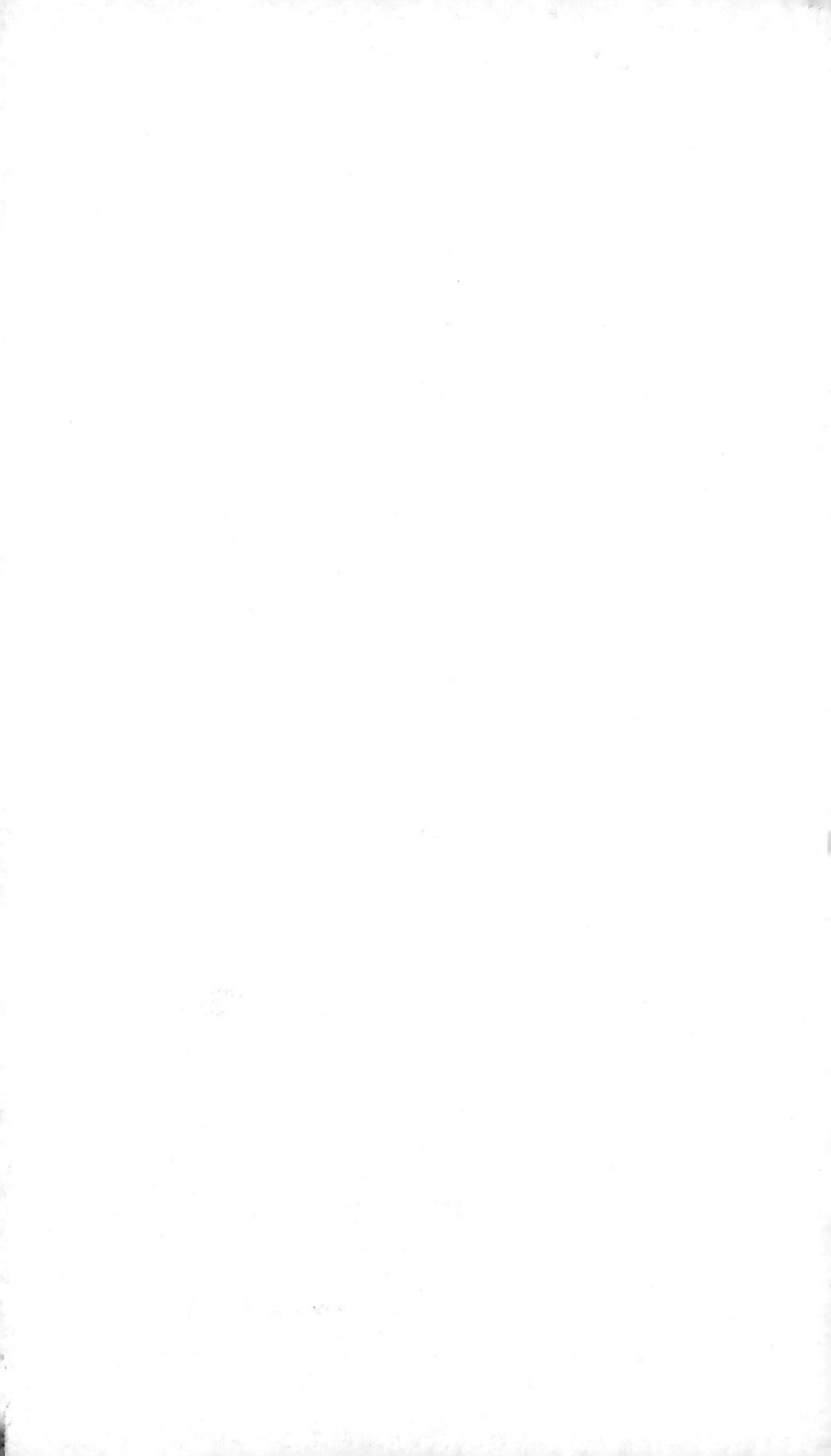

9. Ink on wood: apply oxalic acid.
10. Indelible ink:
    a. If base is aniline dye, it cannot be removed.
    b. If base is silver nitrate, apply a 10 per cent solution of potassium cyanide.
11. Ink eradicator.
12. Dakin's solution, soap, and rubbing.

Rust
1. Use salt and lemon juice, place article in the sun.
2. Apply oxalic acid or dilute hydrochloric acid. Wash out in water.
3. Try salts of lemon.

Fruit
1. Fresh fruit stains (except peaches):
    a. Rub stain with salt and apply boiling water.
2. Old fruit stains:
    a. Soak in weak oxalic solution.
    b. Bleach with peroxide and ammonia.
3. Peach stains:
    a. Apply alcohol.
4. Grape juice stains:
    a. Bleachers: Oxalic acid, ammonia, or hydrogen peroxide.

Chocolate and cocoa stains
1. Cover with borax and soak with cold water. ·Pour boiling water through stain.

Coffee and tea stains
1. Ordinary laundering will usually remove stain.
2. Pour on boiling water from a height.
3. Apply dilute ammonia; wash when color disappears.
4. Use peroxide and ammonia for old coffee and tea stains.

Grease
1. Cannot be removed by washing in water.
2. Soak in kerosene before washing.
3. Wash with turpentine; oil may be absorbed by using blotting paper or powdered chalk.
4. Gasoline may be used for materials that cannot be washed.
5. Chloroform may be used. Always use in daylight and in a draft, and have several folds of cloth under stain.
6. Axle grease on linen:
    a. Grease well with lard or butter and wash in tepid, soapy water.
7. Tar:
    a. Use gasoline.

8. Glue:
   a. Soak in vinegar and wash in soapy water.
9. Grass stains:
   a. Soak in alcohol and wash in usual way.
   b. Apply lemon juice and salt and place in the sun.
10. Gum:
   a. Remove with ether.
   b. Alcohol.

Mucus
1. Wash in ammonia and water or in salt and water before using soap.

Perspiration
1. Use a strong soap solution and let article lie in the sun.

Urine
1. Wash with warm, soapy water.
2. Sponge with alcohol.

Feces
1. Wash with cold water at once.
2. Allow to soak in cold, soapy water and boil.

Mildew
1. Moisten with strong soap solution.
2. Apply a paste of soap, salt, and chalk, and leave in strong sunlight for several hours; if unsuccessful, use Javelle water or other bleaching agent.
3. Try lemon juice and salt.

References
Harmer, *Principles and Practice of Nursing*, pp. 45–47.

Removal of Stains from Drugs

Coal-tar products
1. Try tincture of green soap.
2. Try potassium permanganate and oxalic acid.

Argyrol
1. Soak in 10 per cent potassium cyanide.
2. Use Dakin's solution.
3. Bichloride of mercury 1/500; rinse well.

Silver nitrate
1. Bichloride of mercury; rinse well.
2. 5 per cent potassium cyanide.
3. Remove from hands with potassium iodide solution.
4. Remove from linen with argyrol or bichloride of mercury solution 1/500; rinse thoroughly.

Acid stains
1. Neutralize with ammonia.
2. If acid has removed the color, it may be brought back with chloroform.
3. For a skin burn with acid, rinse with water immediately, to dilute the acid, and apply ammonia.
4. In case of a phenol (carbolic acid) burn, apply alcohol at once.

Iodine
1. On linen:
   a. Fresh stains may be removed by washing in warm, soapy water.
   b. May be removed by boiling.
2. On wood:
   a. Cover with cold-starch paste until iodine is absorbed and wash with ammonia and water.
3. On skin:
   a. Wash with alcohol.

Potassium iodide
1. Dakin's solution.
2. Alcohol.
3. Hot ammonia.

Potassium permanganate
1. Oxalic acid solution.
2. Hydrogen peroxide.

Oil
1. On linen:
   a. Use kerosene, then soap and water.
   b. Camphorated oil is removed with ether.
   c. Try turpentine on carron oil.
2. On marble:
   a. Wash with sodium bicarbonate solution.
   b. Apply paste of ammonia and whiting and let stand for 24 hours.

Paint
1. Try benzine or turpentine. (If dry, apply vaseline first.)

Bichloride of mercury
1. Soak in Labarraque's solution for several hours, then wash and rinse.

Balsam
1. Alcohol.
2. Bleachers.

Picric acid
  1. Dakin's solution.

Mercurochrome
  1. Dakin's solution.
  2. Soap and water and rub.

Cod-liver oil
  1. Carbon tetrachloride, followed by soap and water.
  2. Acetone.

Extract of Hamamelis
  1. Use a good bleach—for example, Javelle water.
  2. Soap and water.

Tincture of benzoin
  1. Javelle water.
  2. Ammonia.
  3. Hydrogen peroxide.
  4. Alcohol.
  5. Ether.

References
  Goostray and Karr, *Chemistry for Nurses*, pp. 123–27.
  Bogert, *Fundamentals of Chemistry*, p. 328.

Care of Rubber Goods

Purpose
  1. To prolong life of articles.
  2. To put articles away ready for use when needed.

Articles in common use in hospital
  Gastric lavage tube.
  Ewald evacuating bulb.
  Rehfuss tubes.
  Ear bulb.
  Rubber gloves.
  Hard rubber goods (enema and douche tips, bougies, syringes, pessaries, catheters).
  Rectal and colon tubes.
  Rubber and silk catheters.
  Silk ureter catheters.
  Rubber rings.
  Hot-water bags, icecaps, and ice collars.
  Rubber sheets and mackintoshes.
  Rubber pillowcases.
  Rubber aprons.
  Kelly pads.
  Rubber protectors.

General instructions

Rubber appliances are expensive and need constant attention.
1. Never stick pins into a rubber appliance.
2. Oil and grease cause rubber to soften and partially dissolve.
3. Acids corrode it.
4. Prolonged heat destroys it.
5. Folding cracks it. All rubber sheeting should be rolled or hung on bars.
6. If not used, it becomes dry; it should be soaked in cold water occasionally.
7. See that rubber washer is on stopper and cap of hot-water bottle. (Caps, stoppers, and rings may be ordered when lost.)
8. Hot-water bottle stoppers can be attached to container with tape or string if necessary.
9. Clamps on rubber tubing should always be unfastened when not in use; drain well and coil loosely, never at sharp angles.

To mark

1. Use fresh stick of lunar caustic, slightly moistened, if there is no other provision.

Care of Ewald evacuating tube, gastric lavage tube, Rehfuss tube, and ear bulb

1. Clean immediately after use, with cold water, allowing plenty of cold water to run through tube.
2. Wash in warm, soapy water and rinse.
3. Drop into boiling water for 3 minutes. Do not leave until you have removed tube and bulb.
4. Remove, rinse in cold water, dry thoroughly, and put away, being sure that the tubing is not bent.

Care of rubber gloves

1. Clean immediately after use with cold water.
2. Wash in warm, soapy water and rinse.
3. Dry thoroughly.
4. Inflate gloves to discover holes and put aside all imperfect ones.
5. Powder.

Care of hard rubber goods

1. Clean with cold water immediately after use.
2. Wash with warm, soapy water and rinse.
3. Keep in bichloride of mercury 1/1000 or, if not being used daily, in dry container.

Care of rectal and colon tubes and catheters

1. Clean with cold water immediately after use, allowing plenty of cold water to run through tube.

2. Wash with warm, soapy water and rinse. Be sure that tube is *clean before boiling.* Use applicator if necessary.
3. Drop into boiling water for 3 minutes.
4. Remove, rinse in cold water and dry, and put away in container provided for them.

Care of silk catheters
1. Clean with cold water immediately after use, allowing plenty of cold water to run through the catheter.
2. Wash with warm, soapy water and rinse.
3. Place in solution of bichloride of mercury 1/1000, or oxycyanide of mercury.

Care of rubber rings, hot-water bags, icecaps, ice collars, and Kelly pads
1. Wash with warm, soapy water and dry.
2. Slightly inflate and put in place provided for them.

Care of rubber sheets, mackintoshes, pillowcases, aprons, and protectors
1. Wash with warm, soapy water and dry.
2. Hang in place provided for them.

When put away
1. All rubber should be dry.
2. Tubing should be straight.
3. Bags, air cushions, ice bags, etc., should be slightly inflated.
4. Gloves should be powdered.

References
Harmer, *Principles and Practice of Nursing,* pp. 360–62.
Kelley, *Textbook of Nursing Technique,* pp. 66–68.
"Misuse of Rubber Goods," *American Journal of Nursing,* 1931, p. 1071.

Care of Glassware

Purpose
1. To prolong life of articles.
2. To put articles away ready for use when needed.

Articles in common use in hospital

Connecting and irrigating tips.	Murphy drip.
Catheters.	Medicine droppers.
Douche points.	Glass funnels.
Syringes.	Glass graduates.

Procedure
1. Clean in cold water immediately after use.
2. Wash with warm, soapy water and rinse. Be sure that glass is *clean before boiling.* Use cotton applicator if necessary.

3. Wrap and put into warm water (never boiling), bring to boiling point, and boil for 2 minutes.
4. Remove carefully, dry, and put away in place provided for them.

Care of the Linen Room

Purpose
1. To have the linen as conveniently placed as possible and in order at all times.

Articles in common use in the hospital

Linen.	Rubber sheets.
Blankets.	Rubber pillowcases.
Pillows.	

Procedure
Linen shelves are washed weekly.
1. Linen:
   a. Have a definite place for each piece of linen.
   b. Place all pieces uniformly on the shelves with the fold to the front.
   c. Put aside all articles to be mended or exchanged.
2. Blankets:
   a. Fold from top to bottom and then fold in half again.
   b. Then fold ends to center with strips on the inside.
   c. Place in space provided for them with the fold to the front.
3. Rubber sheets and rubber pillowcases:
   a. Roll or hang on poles provided for them.
4. Pillows:
   a. Pile neatly on the shelf.

References
Harmer, *Principles and Practice of Nursing*, pp. 50–51.
Kelley, *Textbook of Nursing Technique*, p. 27.
Southard, *Institutional Administration*, pp. 118–22.

Care and Arrangement of Flowers *

Flowers are a "thrill of encouragement and a will to live" to the weary hearts of the sick and as such should be accorded the same respectful attention as medicines and treatments.

If the life of these beautiful messages of hopefulness and love is shortened and they are made unsightly by improper treatment, their proper mission is entirely defeated. Nothing more than a few minutes of interested attention and some simple rules are necessary for the care of hospital flowers.

* Irene V. Kelley, *Textbook of Nursing Technique*, p. 27.

Points to be remembered

1. Keep all flowers out of direct drafts.
2. The freshest flowers will soon languish in vases that are too small for their length of stem, and only half filled with water.
3. Flowers crowded too tightly not only droop quickly but lose half their beauty by the loss of their natural grace and charming pose.
4. Always use deep, roomy bowls or vases, with water enough to cover the stems a little more than half their length.
5. If a deep enough bowl is not available, dampen a newspaper heavily and wrap around the stems. Insert flowers, paper and all, into the small bowls filled with water. The papers will keep the stems moist and the flowers fresh.
6. In the case of arranged baskets of cut flowers, be sure that the receptacle contains sufficient water.
7. Water potted plants and change the water on cut flowers daily.
8. It will prolong the life of cut flowers to clip a little from the stems every day.
9. Flowers should be removed from patient's room at night.

Care of flower room

1. Wash shelves and sink with soap and water.
2. Leave room in order after arranging flowers.

References

Hall, "Care and Arrangement of Flowers," *American Journal of Nursing,* 1932, p. 16.

Ruedel, "Care of Cut Flowers," *American Journal of Nursing,* 1933, pp. 832–34.

Kelley, *Textbook of Nursing Technique,* p. 27.

The Serving of Food to the Sick

Purpose

1. To nourish the sick.

General instructions

1. Follow the doctor's orders.
2. Before serving tray, remove medicine glasses, emesis basins, etc., from bedside table and place tray in convenient position for patient to reach.
3. See that patient is in a comfortable position before being served.
4. Have tray clean, neatly set, conveniently arranged, and as attractive as possible.
5. Serve food promptly.
6. Serve hot foods hot on hot dishes.

a. See that steam table is turned on 15 minutes before serving food and that dishes to be warmed are put in warming oven.

b. If tray is taken to patient while a treatment is being given, take food back to kitchen and see that food is kept hot.

c. Serve convalescing patients first and helpless patients last.

7. Serve cold foods cold on cold dishes.
8. Avoid serving greasy, overdone, or underdone food.
9. Do not serve too many varieties at a time; for example, liquid diet: tea and soup.
10. Keep patient in a cheerful frame of mind.
11. Use diplomacy rather than force in getting patient to take food.
12. Do not hurry the patient.
13. Do not serve the dishes too well filled; a second serving is preferable.
14. Encourage the patient to masticate the food well.
15. Cut meat for patient if he is unable to do so himself.
16. Serve food to very sick patients often, and in small quantities.
17. Consider the preferences of the patient in serving and seasoning food.
18. In carrying liquids to a patient in a cup or glass, always carry on small tray or saucer.

Feeding a patient who is in a reclining position

1. Protect patient's gown and bed with a napkin or towel. Dry mouth with napkin as necessary.
2. In giving liquids, pour a small quantity into a cup, raise the head slightly by slipping arm and hand under pillow. If head is raised too far forward, it makes it difficult for patient to swallow.
3. Drinking tubes are preferable to lifting the head unless patient is too weak to draw fluid through a tube. Always clean a tube at once after it has been used.
4. Never use a glass tube in feeding a delirious or unconscious patient. Pass the spoon back in the mouth, pressing the tongue gently with the spoon, and the food will generally be swallowed. Carry only a small amount of food in the spoon and do not feed too fast. A rubber ear syringe or medicine dropper can be used to feed a patient if other means fail.
5. The nurse should be seated at bedside, if possible, while feeding patient.

Nourishment dishes

1. The nurse is responsible for dishes and utensils used for nourishment.

2. Dishes are to be collected from bedside and washed immediately after use.

Glass drinking tubes
1. Do not let fluids dry in them.
2. Rinse in cold water immediately after use.
3. Wash with soapy water, using special brush.
4. Boil in sodium bicarbonate solution (1 dram to 1 qt. of water).
5. Rinse thoroughly in warm water and dry.
6. Place in container.

Nurses are not permitted to eat in diet kitchens
1. Food belongs to the patients.
2. Time belongs to the patients.
3. Food is not to be distributed to anyone but patients.

Reference
Harmer, *Principles and Practice of Nursing*, pp. 114–35.

II. FOR THE COMFORT OF THE PATIENT

Purpose
1. To make and keep the patient comfortable.

General instructions
1. Never discuss a patient's condition in his presence, even if he is unconscious.
2. Never discuss a patient's condition with another patient.
3. Satisfy the questions of patients, whenever possible, in accordance with good judgment and common sense.
4. Never go out of a room without leaving it in better condition and more pleasant for the patient and with a happier atmosphere than when you entered.
5. Whenever possible, complete a piece of work before starting another.
6. Sources of discomfort:
   a. Bad ventilation and bright light in eyes.
   b. Noise, loud voices, whispering, hard heels, squeaking shoes, leaking faucets, banging doors, squeaking hinges.
   c. Permitting patient to remain in one position too long. Unless otherwise ordered or patient's condition is such that the presence of extensions makes moving quite impossible, he should never remain in one position longer than 6 hours.
   d. Extremes of temperature.
   e. Lack of cleanliness.
   f. Weight and pressure on sensitive parts.
   g. Wrinkled bedding.

References
Harmer, *Principles and Practice of Nursing,* pp. 84–90.
Kelley, *Textbook of Nursing Technique,* pp. 45–46.

The Open Bed *

Purpose
1. Comfort of the patient.
   a. Tight foundation.
   b. Not too tight over feet.
2. Sanitation: bedding not to touch floor or uniform.
3. Economy of time, of linen, of energy.
4. Neat appearance while working and when finished.

Necessary articles
2 large sheets.
Drawsheet.

---

* Moving pictures have been made of this procedure. See Preface, page iv.

19

Spread.

2 pillowcases.

2 pillows (1 small pillow and pillowcase in addition in private rooms).

Rubber drawsheet.

2 wool blankets.

Mattress pad.

Procedure

1. Place chair conveniently at side or at foot of bed.
2. Place necessary clean linen ready for use over head of bed or on chair.
3. Remove cases from pillows, if necessary, and place in hamper bag or on chair.
4. Place pillows flat on chair.
5. Loosen bedding all around, beginning at center top.
6. Fold spread from top to bottom and then in half, and place in hamper bag or hang over back of chair.
7. Fold blankets and top sheet in the same manner.
8. Pick up cotton drawsheet at center of top and bottom, and place in hamper bag or hang over back of chair.
9. Pick up rubber drawsheet in same manner.
10. Fold bottom sheet the same as spreads and blankets, and remove mattress pad.
11. Turn mattress end to end and replace mattress pad.
12. Put on the under sheet right side up with wide hem at the head, allowing 8 inches to tuck under at the head of mattress. Place center of sheet in center of the bed. Unfold all linen on bed and do not shake.
13. Tuck under tight and smooth at head.
14. Fold corner and make an angle of 45 degrees (envelope fold).
15. Tuck in at side to foot of mattress.
16. Place rubber drawsheet across center of bed, upper edge 9 inches from head of mattress.
17. Cover with cotton drawsheet, tucking at least 2 inches, and 4 inches if width of sheet allows, over the edge of rubber drawsheet.
18. Tuck in both drawsheets.
19. Walk around bed, turn back the drawsheets, and repeat steps 13–18.
20. Walk to foot of bed and make envelope corner on each side at foot of mattress.
21. Put upper sheet, wrong side up, with seam of wide hem even with head of mattress.
22. Tuck in foot, making envelope corner.
23. Place first blanket, upper edge 6 inches from head of bed. Fold

upper edge under 3 inches. Fold lower edge under even with edge of mattress and tuck under at side.

24. Put on second blanket, upper edge 9 inches from head of bed. Tuck in at foot, making square corner and tucking under at side.
25. Put on spread, right side up, top edge even with head of mattress, if possible. Be sure it is on evenly and tuck under surplus at foot at least 8 inches. Make envelope corner at side.
26. Turn spread over edge of blankets and sheet down over spread. Turn under hem and make finished fold of 9 inches.
27. Walk around bed; turn loose bedding up on bed. Finish as other side.
28. Make a fold underneath on seam of pillow at head of bed.
29. Place pillow flat, open end of case away from the door.
30. Replace furniture.
31. Remove soiled linen. Leave unit in order.

Note. — This procedure may be varied to include making a bed with no additional clean linen, with an entire change of linen, or with any partial change. When only one sheet is changed, the former upper sheet may be used as the lower sheet.

References
Harmer, *Principles and Practice of Nursing,* pp. 52–57.
Kelley, *Textbook of Nursing Technique,* pp. 21–25.

Modification for a Closed Bed *

1. Fold top sheet back over blankets.
2. Turn under hem and make finished fold of 9 inches.
3. Put on spread, top edge even with head of mattress, and finish bottom the same as for open bed.

The Post-operative Bed †

Purpose
1. Convenience in caring for the patient.
2. Warmth for the patient.
3. Comfort for the patient.
4. Protection for the bed.

Necessary articles

2 face towels.	3 tongue blades.
Spread.	Woolen blanket or bath blanket.
Mattress pad.	Rubber protector 12 inches wide, and
2 large sheets.	long enough to tuck in on both sides
	at head of bed.

* Closed bed is always made after discharge of patient and cleaning of unit or room.
† Moving pictures have been made of this procedure. See Preface, page iv.

2 wool blankets.
2 cotton drawsheets.
Rubber drawsheet.
2 pillows.
2 pillowcases.
Roller bandage.
Pencil and paper.

2 safety pins.
Mouth wipes (cellu-wipes or paper napkins cut in fourths).
Cornucopia or paper bag.
2 kidney basins.
3 hot-water bottles or bed warmer; temperature of water 150° F.

Procedure

1. Strip bed.
2. Turn mattress.
3. Make foundation bed on one side.
4. Place rubber protector across head of bed.
5. Cover with cotton drawsheet folded lengthwise, fold surplus under protector at the bottom, and tuck both under mattress.
6. Walk around bed, complete foundation bed, and tuck rubber protector and drawsheet under mattress at head.
7. Place bath blanket on bed even with top of mattress. Fold back corners at foot to meet in center.
8. Fold top down 12 inches from top of mattress.
9. Fold blanket over on open side even with edge of mattress.
10. Place top covers on bed. Do not tuck in. Finish top in usual way.
11. Make 8-inch fold of all covers even with foot of mattress.
12. Make 8-inch fold on side to be opened.
13. Fold towel over top edge of upper bedding.
14. Tie pillow to head of bed with a bandage.
15. Place hot-water bottles or jugs under the blanket at the top, middle, and bottom of bed. (Never leave hot-water bottles next to patient unless temperature of water conforms to regulation.)
16. Pin paper bag or cornucopia to cotton drawsheet at upper edge of bed.
17. Pin mouth wipes to cotton drawsheet at upper edge of bed.
18. Cover stand with half of face towel, wrong side toward table, and place on it kidney basins, tongue blades, and pencil and paper, and cover with other half of towel.
19. Place chair at foot of bed, and table beyond head or away from bed.
20. When patient returns:
    a. Remove hot-water bottles.
    b. Fold bedding and bath blanket to opposite side of bed.
    c. Place patient in bed.
    d. Cover with bedding.
    e. Wrap patient well in blanket, tucking around shoulders.
    f. Adjust towel under chin.

g. Take pulse.
h. Tuck bedding in at foot and make corners in usual manner.
20. After-care of patient:
   a. Stay with patient and watch pulse closely.
   b. Chart in nurse's remarks column the time of return from Operating Room and general condition. Take pulse and record respiration every 10 minutes for one hour or, if patient is still unconscious, until he regains consciousness.

References
Harmer, *Principles and Practice of Nursing,* pp. 334–41.

To Give and Remove Bedpan and Urinal

Purpose
To place pan comfortably in proper position with minimum amount of exposure.

Necessary articles

Bedpan.	Hand basin.
Bedpan cover.	Urinal and cover.

Preparation of equipment
1. Warm bedpan with hot water, dry, and cover.
2. Carry bedpan, with toilet paper and hand basin of warm water, to bedside.
3. Place pan on chair and hand basin on bedside stand.

Preparation of patient
1. Screen completely.
2. Triangle covers back.
3. Place toilet paper at side of pillow within reach of patient.
4. Hang bedpan cover over side rail bar of bed.
5. Flex the knees.
6. Draw the gown back.

Procedure
1. Place hand under coccyx and place in position.*
2. Place signal light within reach of patient.
3. Leave patient comfortable.
4. When removing bedpan from a female patient, if patient is unable to care for herself, wind several thicknesses of paper around the hand, cleanse and dry rectum. (The orderly cares for the male patient.)
5. Place hand as before and with other hand draw pan down and out. Cover pan as soon as removed.

* When taking a bedpan to a male patient, also take a urinal.

6. If necessary, wash and dry patient's buttocks.
7. Adjust bedclothes.
8. Place hand basin, towel, and soap in position for patient to wash and dry hands.
9. Remove screen.
10. Carry bedpan, toilet paper, and hand basin to service room.

After-care of equipment
1. Observe contents of pan carefully and empty.
2. Rinse pan first in cold water, then cleanse with mop and soapy water.
3. Rinse and replace pan.
4. Wash bedpan mop under running water.
5. Wash and boil hand basin, dry, and replace on shelf.

To give a urinal
1. Warm, dry, cover, and carry to bedside with hand basin of warm water.
2. Lift bedclothes at side of bed and place urinal within reach of patient's hand.
3. Cover the urinal and remove to service room.

References
Harmer, *Principles and Practice of Nursing*, pp. 153–60.

To Fill a Hot-Water Bottle

Purpose
To apply heat with safety and comfort to the patient.

Necessary articles

Hot-water bottle.	Pitcher.
Cover.	Bath thermometer.

General instructions
1. Be sure that bottle is in good condition.
2. Always take temperature of the water with a bath thermometer. *Do not take temperature in any other way.*
3. Expel the air and be sure that bag is not too heavy.

Procedure
1. Fill bottle half full of water at 120° F.
2. Expel the air by folding bottle in half and pressing water to neck of bottle.
3. Screw in cap.
4. Test for leaks by turning bottle upside down.
5. Dry, cover, and apply.

References
Kelley, *Textbook of Nursing Technique*, p. 63.
Harmer, *Principles and Practice of Nursing*, p. 250.

To Fill an Icecap

Purpose
To apply ice with safety and comfort to the patient.

Necessary articles

Icecap.	Cover.
Ice in basin.*	Small pitcher for warm water.

General instructions
1. Be sure that cap is in good condition.
2. Be sure that metal cover fits and has a rubber washer.
3. Be sure that cap is not too heavy.
4. Do not puncture cap with sharp pieces of ice.
5. Always replace cover to prevent cover and washer from being lost.
6. Ice applications must be changed frequently to accomplish their purpose.

Procedure
1. Break the ice into pieces about the size of a walnut.
2. If necessary to take off the sharp edges, pour warm water over the ice.
3. Test cap to see that it does not leak by putting on cover and squeezing bag to see if any air escapes.
4. Fill with ice one-third to one-half full.
5. Expel the air from the bag by drawing top and bottom apart and squeezing sides together as much as possible.
6. Screw on cap and wipe dry.
7. Cover and apply.

After-care of equipment
1. Wash with warm, soapy water and dry.
2. Inflate slightly and put in place provided.

Note. — The above procedure is also used for filling an ice collar. Care should be taken in the application of the latter that it is secure and comfortable for the patient.

References
Kelley, *Textbook of Nursing Technique*, p. 64.
Harmer, *Principles and Practice of Nursing*, pp. 281–82.

* If ice is kept in the kitchen, take a sufficient quantity (but do not waste it) in a basin and take to the service room and fill the icecap.

The Application of Binders

Purpose
1. To keep applications and surgical dressings in place.
2. To make compression.
3. To afford support and comfort to the patient.

General instructions
Carelessly and inefficiently applied binders are worse than none.

Kinds of binders
1. Scultetus or many-tailed binders.
2. Straight binders.
3. T-binders.
4. Hernia or male T-binders.
5. Breast binders.

Procedure
1. Scultetus:
    a. Fanfold binder half way and place under patient so that center of binder will come to center of back.
    b. Draw out on other side.
    c. Apply from below toward chest, folding strips alternately and obliquely, being careful to arrange smoothly and snugly.
    d. Pin binder, placing pins lengthwise. Use as many pins as are necessary to hold binder in place.
2. Straight binder:
    a. Fanfold binder and place under patient in such a way that center of binder will come to center of back.
    b. Draw out on other side.
    c. Fold ends of binder until it just meets over largest part of body.
    d. Pin binder down center.
    e. Pin a dart down each side so that binder will fit patient.
3. T-binders for perineum:
    a. Place around patient's waist.
    b. Pin perineal pad to tab at back and front of binder, or bring the strip attached to back of straight band that encircles the waist up over perineum to hold dressings in place.
    c. Pin to binder in front, being careful that pad is in place and strap not too tight.
4. Hernia binder adjusted same as T-binder.
5. Breast binder:
    a. Fanfold binder and place under patient so that center of binder will come to center of back.

b. Draw out on other side.

c. Place breasts in proper position away from axillae.

d. Pin from lower edge of binder to upper edge.

e. Pin straps over shoulder.

f. Pin a dart down each side, if necessary, for fitting of binder.

References

Kelley, *Textbook of Nursing Technique*, pp. 70–71.

Harmer, *Principles and Practice of Nursing*, pp. 284–89.

To Change the Gown

THE HOSPITAL GOWN

1. Loosen soiled gown.
2. Draw off one sleeve, slip clean gown underneath soiled one, covering chest.*
3. Put on sleeve by crushing together so that patient's hand can be grasped through opening.
4. Draw over arm and shoulder.
5. Remove other sleeve.
6. Finish putting on gown and tie strings.

THE LONG, CLOSED GOWN

To remove soiled gown

1. Loosen about neck.
2. Flex patient's knees.
3. Bring lower part of gown up close to buttocks.
4. Slip hand underneath back, just below waist.
5. Raise buttocks at the same time with other hand, slipping gown to waist.
6. Raise head and shoulders as in changing pillows, with other hand draw gown about shoulders.
7. Remove one sleeve, then raise head and slip gown off over head; remove other sleeve.

To put on gown

1. Crush together back of gown.
2. Put on one sleeve, crush as with hospital gown.
3. Raise head and slip gown over head.
4. Slip other arm into gown.
5. Raise head and shoulders, draw gown to waist.
6. With knees flexed raise body by placing hand under back, below waist.
7. With other hand draw gown below hips, then down over legs and ankles.

* Draw off sleeve nearest you first, or, if patient has injured arm, draw off sleeve from uninjured arm first.

To Replace Upper Bedclothes with a Bath Blanket

Procedure
1. Fold bath blanket crosswise.
2. Fold open edges back to fold, one on each side.
3. Place blanket folded with open edge across chest of patient toward head of bed.
4. Have patient hold the lower open edge or tuck it securely around his shoulders.
5. Face foot of bed and grasp the other open edge between fourth and fifth fingers.
6. Grasp upper covers between thumb and other two fingers.
7. Fanfold the covers to foot of bed.

To Change Pillows

To remove
1. Slip one arm under head, with hand under far shoulder blade; raise patient slightly.
2. With one hand remove pillow by drawing it out from opposite side of bed, then place it on side of bed and remove arm from under the head.

To replace
1. Place pillows at far side of bed.
2. Support patient as above.
3. With free hand draw pillow under head.
4. Avoid arranging pillows exactly on top of each other under patient's head. Try to fit the curve of neck and shoulders.

Evening Care *
(Time of Care Depending on Hospital Routine)

Purpose
1. To make the patient comfortable.

Necessary articles

Basin of warm water.	Cup with mouthwash.
Toilet articles.	Drinking tube if necessary.
Kidney basin.	Necessary linen.

Preparation of equipment
1. Prepare necessary articles and carry to bedside.

Preparation of patient
1. Screen completely if in a ward; if in a room, place screen before door.†
2. Arrange articles ready for use. Place clean linen in order over head of bed or on chair.

---

* Moving pictures have been made of this procedure. See Preface, page iv.
† Give the patient a bedpan at this time if she desires it.

3. Fanfold top bedding down and replace with bath blanket.

Procedure

1. Care of the mouth and teeth:
   a. Place a towel and kidney basin under patient's chin.
   b. Put toothpaste on the brush and pour water over it. If patient is unable to brush his teeth, gums, and tongue, the nurse will do it for him.
   c. Follow brushing by rinsing of mouth with mouthwash.
   d. Remove kidney basin and towel.
2. Remove pillows under head, extra pillows, rubber rings, etc.
3. Remove binder and place over back of chair.
4. Remove gown and place over back of chair.
5. Care of face and hands:
   a. Protect bath blanket with face towel.
   b. Wash eyes before using soap and then wash face and neck, using soap if desired, and dry.
   c. Place towel on bed under patient's arm and hand.
   d. Put basin on towel and place patient's hand in basin and wash.
   e. Dry the hand.
   f. Repeat the procedure for the other hand, transferring basin to other side of bed.
6. Care of the back:
   a. Turn patient on side, face away from you.
   b. Spread bath towel on bed lengthwise, with one edge next to patient's back.
   c. Expose, wash, and dry upper half of back, beginning at the hair line; then cover with bath blanket and wash and dry lower half.
   d. Put alcohol in palm of hand and rub entire back until dry. Rub with long downward strokes and a rotary motion, rotating outward from the spine. Work evenly and smoothly, with a firm, gentle, and effective touch. Hands must be smooth, warm, and dry. Avoid jerking or jarring the patient.
   e. Shake powder into hands and dust back lightly.
   f. Brush out crumbs with bath towel and tighten foundation bed. Put on a fresh drawsheet if necessary.
   g. Replace one sleeve of gown.
   h. Fanfold binder into place.
   i. Turn patient toward you and finish cleansing and rubbing of back, shoulders, and hips.
   j. Finish putting on gown.
7. Walk around bed and complete brushing out crumbs and tightening of foundation bed. Tie gown.

8. Pull binder out.
9. Turn patient on back and pull up mattress.
10. Walk around bed and fasten binder.
11. Replace pillows. Place face towel under head and comb hair. Remove face towel.
12. As bath blanket is removed, pull up upper bedclothes and straighten. Fold bath blanket and put in place provided for it.
13. Straighten corners.

After-care of patient
1. See that patient has fresh water and an extra blanket if necessary.
2. Attend to any other requests of patient.
3. Remove screen.
4. Remove articles and leave room or ward in order.

After-care of articles
1. Clean, replace, and put in proper places.

Record
1. Hour, condition of patient, and anything unusual.

References
Kelley, *Textbook of Nursing Technique*, pp. 39–40, 57.
Harmer, *Principles and Practice of Nursing*, pp. 143–51.

To Keep a Patient from Slipping Down in Bed *

Articles needed
Pillow and bandage or knee roll.
Rubber pillowcase.
Large sheet.

Procedure
Method no. 1. If pillow is used:
1. Cover with rubber case, roll, and fasten with bandage.
2. Fold sheet diagonally and, beginning at the folded corners, roll pillow in it.
3. Triangle covers back.
4. Flex knees and slip roll under knees.
5. Place open part of roll away from patient's body.
6. Fasten on the sides to spring or to head of bed with the corners of the sheet.
Method no. 2:
1. Using one large sheet, fold diagonally 10–12 inches wide.
2. Slip below patient's feet and bring one end to either side of bed and tie to springs or head of bed.

* Moving pictures have been made of this procedure. See Preface, page iv.

Morning Care *

Purpose
1. Comfort.
2. Cleanliness.
3. Neatness.

Necessary articles

Basin of warm water.
Toilet articles.
Kidney basin.

Cup with mouthwash.
Drinking tube, if necessary.
Necessary linen.

Preparation of equipment
1. Prepare necessary articles and carry to bedside.

Preparation of patient
1. Screen completely, if in a ward; if in a room, place screen before door.†
2. Arrange articles ready for use. Place clean linen in order over head of bed or on chair.

Procedure
1. Loosen upper bedding all around by starting on side of bed opposite table.
2. Fold spread from top to bottom and then in half and place in hamper or over back of chair.
3. Fold top blanket the same as spread, and place over back of chair.
4. Place bath blanket over patient and remove second blanket and top sheet. Fold like spread. (If only one sheet is to be changed, top sheet should be saved to replace the bottom one.)
5. Care of the mouth and teeth:
   a. Place a towel and kidney basin under patient's chin.
   b. Put toothpaste on brush and pour water over it. If patient is unable to brush his teeth, gums, and tongue, the nurse will do it for him.
   c. Follow brushing by rinsing of mouth with mouthwash.
   d. Remove kidney basin and towel.
6. Remove pillows under head, extra pillows, rubber rings, etc.
7. Remove binder and place over back of chair or in hamper.
8. Remove gown and place over back of chair or in hamper.
9. Care of the face and hands:
   a. Protect bath blanket with face towel.
   b. Wash eyes before using soap and then wash face, neck, and ears, using soap if desired, dry.

* Moving pictures have been made of this procedure. See Preface, page iv.
† Give patient a bedpan at this time if she desires it.

c. Place towel on bed under patient's arm and hand.

d. Put basin on towel and place patient's hand in basin and wash.

e. Dry the hand.

f. Repeat the procedure for the other hand, transferring basin to other side of bed.

10. Care of the back:

a. Turn patient on side, face away from you.

b. Spread bath towel on bed lengthwise, with one edge next to patient's back.

c. Expose, wash, and dry upper half of back, beginning at hair line; then cover with bath blanket and wash and dry lower half.

d. Put alcohol in palm of hand and rub entire back until dry. Rub with long downward strokes and a rotary motion, rotating outward from the spine. Work evenly and smoothly, with a firm, gentle, and effective touch. Hands must be smooth, warm, and dry. Avoid jerking or jarring patient.

e. Shake powder into hands and dust back lightly.

f. Fold towel and place on head of bed.

11. To change linen:

a. Fanfold the drawsheet close to patient.

b. Fanfold the rubber sheet close to patient.

c. Fanfold the under sheet close to patient.

d. Straighten mattress pad and brush off crumbs.

e. Put on clean under sheet — or top sheet may be used, fanfolding the surplus at center — and tuck in as for foundation bed.

f. Draw rubber sheet into place, being sure that rubber is regulation distance from top of mattress.

g. Put on clean cotton drawsheet, fanfolding the surplus at center.

h. Fold cotton drawsheet 2–4 inches over top of rubber sheet, and tuck both in at side.

i. Fanfold one-half of binder next to patient.

j. Replace one sleeve of gown.

k. Turn patient toward you and finish washing and rubbing of back, shoulders, and hips. Give perineal care if patient is a woman; if a man, the orderly gives it when patient is unable to do it himself.

l. Finish putting on gown.

m. Walk around bed and loosen rest of foundation bed.

n. Fold cotton drawsheet to center and remove, pulling clean sheet and binder into place.

o. Fold back cotton and rubber drawsheets.

   p. Fold under sheet to center and remove, pulling clean sheet into place.

   q. Straighten mattress pad.

   r. Finish foundation bed except foot. Tie gown.

   s. Turn patient on back and pull up mattress.

12. Walk around bed and fasten binder.
13. Replace pillows.
14. Put towel under the head and comb the hair. (Do not neglect to do this.)
15. Remove soiled linen, wash basin, toilet articles, etc.
16. Finish foot of bed.
17. Replace covers, making a finished fold of 9 inches of sheet over spread.
18. To make bed without change of linen:

   a. Loosen foundation bed.

   b. Brush cotton drawsheets free from crumbs with bath towel and fold drawsheet close to patient.

   c. Repeat step b for rubber drawsheet.

   d. Repeat step c for under sheet.

   e. Straighten mattress pad and brush free from crumbs.

   f. Repeat step e for mattress.

   g. Straighten and tuck in lower sheet.

   h. Straighten rubber sheet, being sure that sheet is regulation distance from head of mattress.

   i. Straighten cotton drawsheet, folding 2–4 inches over rubber sheet at the top and tucking both in at the side.

   j. Fanfold half of binder next to patient.

   k. Replace one sleeve of gown.

   l. Turn patient toward you and finish washing and rubbing of back, shoulders, and hips. Give perineal care if patient is a woman; if a man, the orderly gives this when patient is unable to do it himself.

   m. Finish putting on gown.

   n. Walk around bed.

   o. Repeat steps a–i inclusive.

   p. Pull binder out. Tie gown.

   q. Turn patient on back and pull up mattress.

19. Proceed the same as for steps 12–17.

After-care of patient

1. Attend to any request of patient.
2. Remove screen and leave unit complete and in order.

After-care of articles

1. Clean, replace, and put in proper places.

Record
  1. Hour, condition of patient, and anything unusual.

References
  Kelley, *Textbook of Nursing Technique*, pp. 30–33, 56.
  Harmer, *Principles and Practice of Nursing*, pp. 103–05.

To Move a Patient in Bed

Moving a patient from one side of the bed to the other
  1. Flex patient's knees.
  2. Place one arm under patient's neck and shoulders, supporting his head on upper arm.
  3. Place other arm well under patient's back on the opposite side.
  4. Draw upper part of body toward edge of bed.
  5. Slip one hand under lower part of back and the other on the opposite side under the hips.
  6. Draw lower part of body toward edge of bed.
  7. To relieve tension on muscles of the abdomen, flex the knees and support by means of a rubber-covered pillow.
  8. To relieve tension on muscles of back, slip a small pillow under small of back.

Turning a patient on his side
  1. Stand at the side of bed toward which patient is to be turned.
  2. Place arms over patient's body and slip one hand under shoulders and the other under hip.
  3. Gently but firmly roll patient toward you. Make sure he is lying squarely, comfortably on shoulder and hip. The lower leg shoud be extended and the upper flexed and resting on the bed.
  4. If patient is to be left on the side, the hips should be moved toward center of bed.
  5. A pillow may be placed lengthwise at patient's back and one against abdomen if desired, tucked close for support.
  6. A small pillow may be placed between the knees.

Turning a patient with a drawsheet
  1. Patient must be near center or farther side of bed.
  2. Grasp ends of drawsheet from far side of bed and turn patient toward you.
  3. Support patient as previously instructed.

The Use of Mechanical Devices

Purpose
  To make a patient comfortable by means of various mechanical devices.

Kinds of devices
Back-rest.
Bed cradle.
Knee rolls.
Rubber rings.
Cotton rolls.
Sandbags.
Fracture beds.
Electric bakers and electric lights.

THE REMOVABLE BACK-REST *

Purpose
To get patient upon a back-rest with the least possible exertion and to make him comfortable in that position.

Necessary articles
Two or more pillows.
Back-rest.
Knee roll.
Large sheet.
Drawsheet.

Procedure
1. Prepare knee roll.
2. Bring articles to bedside.
3. Place extra pillows on table at right side of bed.
4. Place knee roll on chair, and stand back-rest near foot of bed.
5. Fold upper covers to waistline.
6. Slip arm under pillows and move head and shoulders of patient with pillows over toward right side of bed.
7. Take back-rest around to farther side of bed and set it up in position (an angle of about 60°); cover with drawsheet, placing lengthwise fold at top of back-rest. Place back-rest as near center of bed as possible.
8. Return to right side of bed.
9. Slip left arm under patient's head and right shoulder. Support patient with right arm in front of his chest and over left shoulder. If he is weak, let him lean over that arm, resting head on nurse's shoulder.
10. With left hand, remove pillows from bed and place on table.
11. Reach across and draw back-rest into place.
12. Place first pillow well down at foot of back-rest.
13. Place second pillow above it.
14. If more pillows are used, make patient comfortable by filling in hollow places. Lean patient back on pillows. Arrange drawsheet, go to opposite side and arrange drawsheet.

* Moving pictures have been made of this procedure. See Preface, page iv.

Note. — Two nurses are necessary if patient is too ill to sit up without support.

BED CRADLES (FRAME MADE OF WIRE, IRON, WOOD, OR WICKER)

Purpose
To prevent bedclothes from resting on tender parts.

Necessary articles
Cradle.
Bath blanket.

Procedure
1. Cover patient with bath blanket.
2. Place cradle over injured part.
3. Arrange bedding neatly over frame with box parts at side.
4. Remove bath blanket unless needed for warmth.
5. Keep part warm by using extra blankets over the frame.

Note. — Barrel staves cut in two and covered with gauze may be used as a bed cradle. A box with the ends removed serves the same purpose. A wide board placed at the foot of bed may be used to elevate bedclothes.

KNEE ROLLS

Purpose
To relieve abdominal tension and promote comfort by relaxing muscles.

Necessary articles
Pillow or knee roll.
Rubber slip.
Pillowcase.

Procedure
1. Cover a pillow with a rubber pillowslip.
2. Cover with a pillowcase and make into a roll.
3. Flex patient's knees and slip roll under.

RUBBER RINGS

Purpose
To relieve pressure.

Necessary articles
Rubber ring.
Pillowslip.

Procedure
1. Inflate the ring by covering the valve with a layer of gauze and blowing it about one-third full of air.

2. Cover with a pillowslip.
3. Slip under patient as a pillow.
4. Be sure the valve is between patient's limbs.

COTTON ROLL (CALLED THE "DOUGHNUT")

Purpose
To relieve pressure on bony prominences.

Necessary articles
Cotton.
Bandage.

Procedure
1. Cut a square of cotton.
2. Roll it diagonally and make it into a ring of the desired size.
3. Wrap it firmly with gauze bandaging.
4. Slip under any bony prominence or between patient's knees or ankles. It is sometimes used under patient's ears or heels.
5. If patient is restless, fasten in place by bandage.

SANDBAGS

Purpose
To keep a part immobile or as a support or foundation for other appliances. (They are made of rubber or heavy ticking and filled with sand.)

Necessary articles
Sandbag.
Towel or small pillowcase.
Bandage.

Procedure
1. Cover sandbag with towel or pillowcase and tie with bandage.
2. If used to avoid foot drop and act as a support, place sandbag at patient's feet and tuck a pillow over each side, making an elevation so that bedclothes do not touch toes.

FRACTURE BEDS

Purpose
To keep mattress from sagging or moving.

Necessary articles
Large perforated board the size of the springs.

Procedure
1. The board or boards are placed under the mattress.
2. The bed is made in the usual manner.

ELECTRIC BAKERS AND ELECTRIC LIGHTS

Purpose
1. To relieve pain and stiffness in inflammatory joints.
2. To stimulate absorption of exudates around joints.
3. To relax tissue and increase blood supply in phlebitis.
4. To abort or to hasten the action in carbunculosis.
5. To relieve pain in fractures.
6. To produce hyperemia in infected wounds.

Necessary articles
Apparatus with electric lights or electric baker.

Procedure
1. Place apparatus or baker over desired area. Be sure that light bulbs conform to regulation regarding size and that apparatus is in good condition.
2. Turn on electricity.
3. Note as often as necessary to see that apparatus is all right.

References
Kelley, *Textbook of Nursing Technique,* pp. 47–48, 61–63.

FOWLER'S POSITION

Purpose
1. Comfort of the patient in some medical diseases.
2. To localize infection in the pelvic cavity, promote drainage, and relieve strain on the abdominal muscles and sutures after surgical operations.

Procedure
1. Place patient so that the trunk is at an angle of 60° or 70° with the horizontal.
2. Support with back-rest and pillows.
3. Flex the knees.
4. Use knee roll and sheet to prevent slipping down in bed.

References
Harmer, *Principles and Practice of Nursing,* p. 672.
Cabot and Giles, *Surgical Nursing,* p. 209.

III. LIFTING AND MOVING THE PATIENT

To Make a Stretcher

Purpose

To protect patient when being transported between departments.

Necessary articles

2 sheets.
Blanket.
Stretcher with rubber pad covered with large sheet.
Pillow with case.

Procedure

1. Having covered pad of stretcher with sheet in the usual way, place open sheet on stretcher even with head of stretcher.
2. Place blanket on sheet 8 inches from the top.
3. Place second sheet on blanket even with head of stretcher.
4. When patient is to be placed on stretcher, fanfold covers to foot of bed and cover patient with a bath blanket (this to be left on).
5. Place patient on stretcher, fold the whole up over the feet and turn up sides over patient, making sure that patient's shoulders are well covered.
6. Make a finished fold down the center so that the whole will present a neat appearance.
7. Only the sheet next to patient needs to be changed between patients.

Note. — The stretcher is to be made up in the above way for all patients who are transported between departments. For patients who are moved from one ward to another, or from ward to dressing room, a blanket covering the patient is sufficient. It is advisable that one stretcher be kept made up according to the above procedure.

To Lift a Patient from a Stretcher to a Bed *

Purpose

1. To lift a patient with the least possible discomfort and strain to patient and to nurses.

Procedure

1. Have bed ready to receive patient.
2. Bring stretcher to bed, placing head of stretcher at foot of bed at an angle of 135°.
3. Three nurses come to the same side of stretcher (inner angle).
4. Drop covers of stretcher.

* Moving pictures have been made of this procedure. See Preface, page iv.

5. First nurse places her hands under the patient's head and shoulders.
6. Second nurse places one arm under back and the other under buttocks.
7. Third nurse places one arm under upper part of legs and the other under lower part of legs.
8. Lift patient in unison, holding him forward and resting on nurses' chests.
9. Together walk along stretcher and bed to proper place.
10. Lower patient to bed gradually.
11. First nurse covers patient and removes stretcher blanket.
12. Second and third nurses remove stretcher.

To Lift a Patient

General instructions

1. In moving or readjusting a patient, always have all articles ready, warm, dry, and in a convenient place.
2. Fold all bedclothes and body clothing so that patient will never be exposed and yet will not be hampered by them.
3. The nurse's feet should be separated, weight evenly distributed.
4. Her knees should be flexed and then straightened as patient is lifted.
5. Always flex the body at the hips; the body does not flex at the small of the back, and if you attempt to bend the back and lift, you strain the muscles of the back unnecessarily.
6. Do not lift patient alone if he is heavy or unmanageable.
7. When lifting a patient, reach beyond the center of weight.
8. Give best support to heaviest parts of body.
9. When lifting, support the framework of the body; do not pull on the muscles and skin nor allow the hands to slip.

To lift a helpless patient up on bed

1. Flex patient's knees.
2. Nurse A slips one arm under patient's head and shoulders and one arm under small of patient's back.
3. Nurse B slips one arm just below Nurse A's and one under thigh.
4. Nurse A gives signal to lift, and both lift at once.

To lift a patient up in bed when he is able to assist

1. Flex patient's knees.
2. Patient puts hand on either of nurse's shoulders, or grasps head of bed.
3. Nurse puts one arm under patient's shoulder and one under thighs.

4. Have patient lift himself by his arms, support himself, and push with his feet.

To lift an injured arm or leg

1. When lifting an injured part, place both hands beneath the injured limb on either side of the injury, and raise slowly and gently.
2. Lift an injured limb at the joints, but do not grasp by the fingers or toes.
3. Never place the hands directly under the injured parts.

To Help a Patient Walk

1. The patient's arm is drawn across the helper's shoulder and the body partially supported by grasping the wrist of that arm. The helper puts his other arm around patient's waist.
2. The helper's arm is put across patient's shoulder with the hand in the opposite axilla. With the other hand the helper grasps the upper arm nearest him.

Reference
Harmer, *Principles and Practice of Nursing*, pp. 90–98.

To Change a Mattress

Purpose
1. To change a mattress with patient in bed.

Necessary articles
Fresh mattress standing at an obtuse angle from foot of bed (right side).

Procedure (Two nurses necessary: Nurse A at right of patient, Nurse B at left)
1. Loosen all covers at head, sides, and foot of bed.
2. Remove top bedding, except one blanket and sheet, in routine way.
3. Remove pillows, replacing by small one if necessary for comfort of patient.
4. Fold upper sheet and blanket over patient to meet in center, folding ends under feet.
5. Fold upper corners of bottom sheet diagonally toward patient, folding center of upper portion over pillow.
6. Roll sides of lower sheet up to patient's body and tie ends of rolls over feet.
7. Nurse A moves patient to right side of bed by drawing his head and shoulders over gently, then his body, pulling on roll of lower sheets.
8. Nurse B pulls mattress to left side of bed until half of the wire

spring is exposed, rolling up edge of mattress slightly and supporting against her body.

9. Nurse A places fresh mattress on exposed springs till it touches other mattress in the middle. She supports slightly turned edge against her body.

10. Nurse A draws patient on to fresh mattress by gently drawing over his head and shoulders, then his body, pulling on the roll of lower sheets.

11. Nurse B removes used mattress from left side of bed and stands it against the table.

12. Nurse B draws fresh mattress into position.

13. Nurse B may be dismissed at this point; she removes used mattress.

14. Nurse A makes up bed in usual manner and removes soiled linen.

References

Harmer, *Principles and Practice of Nursing*, p. 96.

To Turn a Mattress with the Patient in Bed

Purpose

1. To turn the mattress with the patient in bed.

Necessary articles

3 large pillows (including the two on the bed).
Small pillow.

Procedure (Two nurses necessary: Nurse A at right of patient, Nurse B at left)

1. Loosen all covers at head, sides, and foot of bed.

2. Remove top bedding, except one blanket and sheet, in routine way.

3. Remove pillows, replacing by small one if necessary for comfort of patient.

4. Fold upper sheet and blanket over patient to meet in center, folding ends under feet.

5. Fold upper corners of bottom sheet diagonally toward patient, folding center of portion over pillow.

6. Roll sides of lower sheet up to patient's body and tie ends of rolls over feet.

7. Nurse A moves patient to right side of bed by gently drawing over his head and shoulders, then his body, pulling on roll of lower sheets.

8. Nurse B pulls mattress to left side of bed until half the wire springs are exposed, rolling up edge of mattress slightly and supporting against her body.

9. Nurse B supports the mattress, rolling its edge against her

slightly while Nurse A places the 3 large pillows lengthwise on exposed springs.

10. Nurse A draws patient on to the pillows by gently drawing over his head and shoulders, then his body, pulling on roll of lower sheets.
11. Nurse B turns the mattress from top to bottom.
12. Nurses A and B lift patient as before from pillows on to the mattress.
13. Nurse A removes pillows and places them on bedside table while Nurse B supports the mattress.
14. Draw mattress into proper position on the spring.
15. Nurse A makes up bed in usual manner and removes soiled linen.

To Undress a Patient in Bed

Procedure
1. Fanfold covers to foot of bed.
2. Cover bed with 2 bath blankets.
3. Fanfold second blanket to foot of bed.
4. Screen bed. Place patient on bed.
5. Remove shoes.
6. Remove clothing from upper part of body. Protect by pulling up second bath blanket.
7. Remove as many articles as possible at one time.
8. Put on gown.
9. Remove clothing from lower part of body.
10. Place clothing on back of chair.
Note. — When garments cannot be removed whole, rip rather than cut the seams. To remove tight-fitting shirts, remove as closed nightgown. If a portion of the body is injured, remove the clothing from the uninjured side first.
11. Give admission bath, remove bath blankets, and pull up covers.
12. Leave patient comfortable and unit in order.

To Dress a Patient in Bed

1. Have all clothing warm and conveniently placed in the order of use.
2. If garment is closed, roll it from hem to neck, draw on sleeves, slip roll over the head and beneath the shoulders.
3. If the clothing opens all the way down, draw on the sleeve on the side away from you.
4. Turn patient toward you, pull garment well up on his shoulder, and tuck rest of garment closely under his back.

5. Turn patient on back and slightly to opposite side. Draw garment beneath the body, slip on the second sleeve, and adjust. If there is an injury, put the sleeve on the injured side first.
6. To put on stocking, turn the leg of the stocking back over the foot, draw on the foot, then draw up over the leg.

Restraining Patients

Purpose
1. To prevent patients from injuring themselves.
2. To prevent patients from getting out of bed.

General instructions
1. Never restrain patients unless absolutely necessary. Always have a doctor's order before doing so.
2. Make restraint effectual. Careless restraint is worse than none.
3. Prevent any restraint from becoming too tight.
4. Watch for and prevent chafing and pressure sores. Pad wristlets with gauze or cotton and bandaging.
5. If patient is violent, have the assistance of enough persons to hold him.
6. Do not fasten one side of body only but fasten one hand and opposite foot unless the policy of the hospital demands that both hands and both feet be fastened.
7. Never fasten hands to head of bed.
8. The presence of restraints indicates the necessity of careful watching.
9. Be sure that circulation is not interfered with.
10. Watch patient's general condition.
11. Restraint of a patient does not indicate lack of gentle treatment.

Articles used
Side boards.
Sheets.
Handcuffs, anklets, and straps.
Strait-jackets.
Clove hitch.
Restraining sheet.

Procedure
1. Side boards are fastened to sides of bed.
2. Sheets:
   a. Fold two sheets diagonally; place one underneath patient's waist and one over abdomen; twist ends of two sheets together, draw through springs, and tie under springs.
   b. Fold a sheet lengthwise and place across chest of patient,

high up under axillae and low down to feet. Twist ends around bars.

 c. Fold sheet diagonally and place under patient's shoulders, bring ends up under axillae, over shoulders, and under pillow, twist ends together, and tie to bar at head of bed or to bar of bed on opposite side. (Restraint of the lower part of the body is usually necessary.)

3. Handcuffs and anklets:
Should be padded. They are adjustable and they lock with a key. Always keep key in definite place. *Never lose key.*

4. Clove hitch:
With a large triangular bandage or a small sheet folded diagonally, make two loops forming a figure 8 with one end up and the other end down. Put loops together with free ends on inside, pass them over hand or foot, twist ends together, and make knot 12 inches from extremity and tie to ends of bedside. If not properly applied, it will either fail to hold or will shut off the circulation.

References
Kelley, *Textbook of Nursing Technique*, pp. 350–51.
Noyes, *Textbook of Psychiatry*, pp. 271–82.

To Get a Helpless Patient Up into a Chair

Purpose
To get a helpless patient out of bed and into a chair with as little exertion as possible, and to make him comfortable.

Necessary articles
Chair with arms.
2 blankets.
2 pillows.
Small pillow.
3 safety pins.
Patient's robe, stockings, and slippers.
Rubber pillowcase.

Procedure
1. Place chair on the convenient side of bed with back of chair parallel to foot of bed. If wheel chair is used, see that the footrest is up and that the wheels are locked.
2. Place blanket in seat of chair, top edge even with chair arms.
3. Place second pillow, open end down, against back of chair, and the small pillow at top for patient's head.
4. Place one pillow in seat. Cover with rubber pillowcase and cotton case.

5. Fold second blanket in half crosswise and lay across back of chair. (This blanket is not necessary if patient has a robe.)
6. Take patient's pulse.
7. Draw patient to front of bed.
8. Slip on patient's robe and stockings. Place slippers on footstool within reach.
9. Fold bedding to foot of bed.
10. Flex patient's knees.
11. With right arm under patient's head and shoulders, and with left arm under knees, lift patient up and at the same time around into a sitting position with feet hanging over edge of bed.
12. Steady patient for a few seconds.
13. Put on slippers.
14. Standing directly in front of patient with one hand in each axilla, slip patient to his feet and at the same time turn him around with his back to the chair.
15. Seat her gently.
16. Put footboard down in place.
17. Fold bottom of blanket up over patient's feet, and sides of blanket one over the other.
18. Bring upper blanket (if used) together over patient's shoulders and fasten at neck with safety pin. Fasten lower edges of blanket around patient's wrist.
19. Strip bed, turn mattress, and make up bed.
20. Note patient's pulse after he has been up 10 minutes and after he has been put back to bed.
21. Reverse process to get patient back to bed.

References

Kelley, *Textbook of Nursing Technique*, pp. 48–50.
Harmer, *Principles and Practice of Nursing,* pp. 93–95.

IV. PERSONAL HYGIENE OF THE PATIENT

The Cleansing Bath *

Purpose
1. Cleanliness.
2. Comfort of the patient.
3. To quiet the nerves.
4. To stimulate the circulation.

General instructions
1. Temperature of room may be higher, but not lower, than 80°
2. Room should be ventilated, but there should be no draft.
3. Temperature of water, 105°–115° F.
4. Avoid unnecessary exposure or chilling.
5. If patient chills or is exhausted after or during bath, give hot drinks, apply external heat, and allow him to rest.
6. Examine patient during bath for rash, swellings, discolorations, pressure sores, abrasions, and vermin.
7. Chart results of observation.
8. Hold corners of washcloth so they do not drag.
9. Do not leave soap in the water.
10. Always rinse and dry each part thoroughly. Follow with palm of hand to insure drying.

Necessary articles
Linen for changing bed.
Bath blanket.
Kidney basin.
Mouthwash cup.
Bath towel.
Face towel.
Washcloth.
Foot tub or bath basin half full of water 105°–115° F.
Toilet articles.

Preparation of equipment
1. Prepare necessary articles and carry to bedside.

Preparation of patient
1. Screen completely if in a ward; if in a room, place screen before door.†
2. Arrange articles ready for use. Place clean linen over head of bed or on chair ready for use.

* Moving pictures have been made of this procedure. See Preface, page iv.
† Give the patient a bedpan at this time if she desires it.

Procedure

1. Loosen upper bedding all around by starting on side of bed opposite table.
2. Fold spread from top to bottom and then in half and place in hamper or over back of chair.
3. Fold top blanket the same as spread and place over back of chair.
4. Place bath blanket over patient and remove second blanket and top sheet. Fold like spread. (If only one sheet is to be changed, the top sheet should be saved to replace the bottom one.)
5. Care of the mouth and teeth:
   a. Place towel and kidney basin under patient's chin.
   b. Put tooth paste on the brush and pour water over it. If patient is unable to brush his teeth, gums, and tongue, the nurse will do it for him.
   c. Follow brushing by rinsing of mouth with mouthwash.
   d. Remove kidney basin and towel.
6. Remove pillows from under head and extra pillows, rubber rings, etc.
7. Remove binder and place over back of chair or in hamper.
8. Remove gown and place over back of chair or in hamper.
9. Care of face:
   a. Protect bath blanket with face towel.
   b. Wash eyes before using soap; then wash face, using soap if desired.
   c. Dry face.
10. Wash and dry neck and ears.
11. Bathe in following order, exposing only area being washed and beginning in each case on extremities or portion of body farthest from nurse:
    a. Arms. Protect bed with bath towel placed lengthwise.
    b. Hands. Place in basin of water, exercising special care between the fingers.
    c. Chest and axillae. Protect with bath towel and bathe underneath it, giving special care to axillae and under pendulous breasts.
    d. Abdomen. Cover chest with face towel and draw bath blanket down. Place bath towel over abdomen. Bathe underneath the bath towel.
    e. Flex knees.
    f. Wash and dry thighs. Protect bed with bath towel placed lengthwise.
    g. Protect bed with bath towel placed lengthwise across foot of bed. Place tub or basin in position in this manner: Put

arm nearest head of bed under patient's legs and hand under his heels. Put other arm across the tub, grasping it on the far side, and move it forward into position at the same time that you raise the patient's feet and legs from the bed. Put blanket over tub.

h. Allow patient's feet to soak. Patient's fingernails may be cleaned while feet are soaking.

i. Bathe feet and remove tub in following manner: Put arm under legs just as when putting them into the tub. Pull tub toward you and place feet on bath towel.

j. Dry feet and care for toenails.

k. Place tub or basin, soap, washcloth, and towel within reach, place towel under hips, and allow patient to finish bath if able. If not, and it is a woman patient, the nurse finishes it; if it is a man, the orderly finishes it. (The nurse should slip out while the patient is finishing his or her bath.)

l. Take tub or basin to service room; empty, wash, and rinse washcloth; fill tub or basin half full of clean water.

12. Care of the back:

a. Turn patient on side, face away from you.

b. Spread bath towel on bed lengthwise, with one edge next to patient's back.

c. Expose, wash, and dry upper half of back, beginning at hair line; then cover with bath blanket and wash and dry lower half.

d. Put alcohol in palm of hand and rub entire back until dry. Rub with long downward strokes and a rotary motion, rotating outward from the spine. Work evenly and smoothly, with a firm, gentle, and effective touch. Hands must be smooth, warm, and dry. Take care not to jerk or jar patient.

e. Shake powder into hands and dust back lightly.

f. Fold towel and place on head of bed.

13. Make half of foundation bed and put on one sleeve of gown.

14. Turn patient toward you and finish washing and rubbing back, shoulders, and hips.

15. Finish putting on gown.

16. Walk around bed and finish making foundation bed except foot. Tie gown.

17. Turn patient on back and pull up mattress.

18. Walk around bed and fasten binder.

19. Replace pillows.

20. Put face towel under head and comb hair. (Do not neglect to do this.)

21. Remove soiled linen, wash basin, toilet articles, etc.

22. Finish foot of bed.

23. Replace covers, making a finished fold of 9 inches of sheet over spread.

After-care of patient
1. Attend to any request of patient.
2. Remove screen and leave unit complete and in order.

After-care of articles
1. Clean, replace, and put in proper places.

Record
1. Hour.
2. Type of bath.
3. Condition of patient and anything unusual.

References
Cavanagh, *Care of the Body*, pp. 121–43.
Harmer, *Principles and Practice of Nursing*, pp. 105–08.
Kelley, *Textbook of Nursing Technique*, pp. 44–45.
Pyle, *Personal Hygiene*, pp. 52–72.

Bed Sores; Decubitus Ulcer; Pressure Areas

Purpose
1. To use all prophylactic measures possible for prevention of the breaking down of tissues from pressure or malnutrition.
2. To treat pressure areas when they develop so as to cause as rapid growth of new tissues as possible.

Prevention
1. The nurse in her daily care must be very careful to remove crumbs and wrinkles from under the patient.
2. No patient should be allowed to remain in one position longer than 6 hours except by special order of the doctor.
3. Use special precautions in care of incontinent patients, or patients with much discharge of any kind, to keep the bed clean and dry.
4. When rubbing the back give special attention to areas at base of the spine, iliac crests, and shoulders.
5. The use of electric lights over the cast with patient turned on abdomen stimulates circulation and helps to prevent pressure areas. This must be done under a doctor's order, however.
6. Carelessness when removing a bedpan sometimes causes a break in the skin, which helps to cause bed sores. The hand should always be slipped betweeen the hips and the pan before it is removed. Leaving a patient on the bedpan for long periods also causes bruising of the tissues and should be avoided.
7. Rubber rings, cotton rings, and cradles must always be used

when there are persistent reddened or bluish areas over bony prominences.

Treatment

1. Notify charge nurse as soon as a break in the skin or definite symptoms of a pressure sore are noticed.
2. Wash surrounding area thoroughly at least twice a day with warm water and soap.
3. Cleanse area well and remove all sloughing material with applicators dampened with solution made of equal parts of hydrogen peroxide and sterile water.
4. Dry with dry cotton applicators.
5. Apply antiseptic astringent solution; the following may be used if ordered by the doctor.
   a. Tannic acid 30 grains in 200 cc. alcohol 70 per cent. (An aqueous solution may be used if alcohol is too irritating.)
   b. Tincture benzoin with Aristol powder.
6. With the use of pillows and air cushions, keep weight of patient off of areas until healed.
7. If there is much drainage, sterile dressings may be used to cover the area, but do not fasten them on with adhesive. Do not allow them to become wrinkled. Change often enough so that they do not become saturated.
8. Exposure to the atmosphere and sunlight has a stimulating effect on the growth of new tissues.
9. Dry heat in the form of electric lights promotes healing.
10. Ointments and oils of all kinds tend to soften tissues and should be used with extreme caution; it is usually better if they are avoided altogether.
11. Irrigations and hot packs may occasionally be ordered by the doctor, for the therapeutic effect of moist heat. Treatment such as outlined above should be used between these.

Record

1. In treatment and medication column: time, treatment, location.
2. In nurse's remarks column: result of treatment.

References

Kelley, *Textbook of Nursing Technique,* pp. 43–44.
Harmer, *Principles and Practice of Nursing,* pp. 98–102.
Sanders, *Modern Methods in Nursing,* pp. 77–82.

To Assist with a Tub Bath

Purpose

1. Comfort.
2. Cleanliness.

General instructions

1. Have bathroom temperature not lower than 80° F.
2. If a patient feels faint when in the tub, let water out of tub, lower the head, and cover patient with a blanket.
3. Do not try to lift a heavy body out of tub.
4. Assist patient to avoid slipping when stepping out of tub.
5. Never allow a weak or very sick patient or a mental case to take a tub bath unassisted.
6. Never turn on hot water faucet when patient is in tub.
7. Do not leave patient in tub of water longer than 10 minutes, unless special orders to the contrary are given.
8. Orderly will assist male patient.
9. Patients with elevated temperatures, cardiac patients, and obstetrical patients are never given a tub bath.
10. Never give a patient a tub bath without permission from the head nurse.

Necessary articles

Bath robe.
Bath blanket.
Gown.
Slippers.
2 bath towels.
Face towel.
Washcloth.
Soap.
Chair at side of tub, covered with bath blanket.

Procedure

1. Prepare room and fill tub half full of water.
2. Take patient to bathroom in wheel chair if she is unable to walk. If patient prefers, or if she is weak, the teeth may be brushed and the face washed while in bed.
3. Assist patient to undress, avoiding exposure.
4. Place bath towel in bottom of tub to minimize possibility of slipping as patient steps into and out of tub.
5. Walk to tub with patient and, standing directly back of her, loosen and hold up bathrobe or bath blanket about her until she steps into tub.
6. Bath towel may be draped around patient's hips to avoid exposure while in tub.
7. Assist patient in washing back.
8. Observe any abnormalities about body.
9. Assist patient in wiping back before she gets out of tub.
10. Hold blanket up about her while she steps out of tub.
11. Dry thoroughly with bath towel.

After-care of patient
1. Assist back into bed.

After-care of articles
1. Soap and towels are left at patient's bedside table.
2. Rinse and wash tub; leave clean and dry.
3. Leave bathroom in order.

Record
1. Time of bath.
2. Any abnormalities noted.
3. Effect of bath.

References
Harmer; *Principles and Practice of Nursing,* pp. 75–80.
Kelley, *Textbook of Nursing Technique,* pp. 57–58.

Care and Hygiene of the Mouth

Purpose
1. To maintain the same hygienic conditions in the mouth as are imperative to maintain in other parts of the patient's body.
2. To prevent deleterious effects of systemic illness on the mucous membranes of the mouth and teeth.

Time
1. Daily, with morning and evening care.
2. Patients who are very ill must, in addition, have their mouths properly cleansed before and after each feeding.

General instructions
1. *Always* wash hands before and after cleansing a patient's mouth.
2. Use fresh solution and clean sponges for each cleansing.
3. Never dip sponge in solution a second time.
4. Be gentle; do not injure mucous membrane.
5. Be sure that your patient *knows how* to carry out oral hygiene procedure *properly* if he does it himself. If he does not *know how*, teach him the proper method *accurately*.
6. Keep toothbrush where it will dry out between cleansings. If possible, have enough brushes so that one brush is used only once a day. (Toothbrush is usually kept in a washable bag in a container in stand or in bathroom.)

Necessary articles
Kidney basin.
Toothbrush.
Dentifrice.
Towel.
Mouthwash solution in cup.

Procedure
1. With patients who are able to carry out oral hygiene procedure themselves:
   a. Give patient articles necessary. (Patient who goes to bathroom needs only brush and dentifrice.)
   b. Observe carefully to ascertain whether he *knows how.*
   c. Instruct him if necessary.
   d. At bedside provide cup of mouthwash solution and an emesis basin.
   e. Provide patient with a towel. The one used for the toilet may be used.
2. Care of helpless patient:
   a. Wash your hands.
   b. Arrange necessary articles.
   c. Place towel across patient under chin.
   d. Place kidney basin under chin.
   e. Put dentifrice on brush.
   f. Have patient separate the teeth enough to relax the mouth.
   g. Place brush with the bristles toward the cutting edge of the teeth.
   h. Then turn with a slow, sweeping motion.
   i. This cleans and at the same time stimulates the gums and cleans the surfaces of the interproximal spaces of the teeth.
   j. Rinse brush frequently while working.
   k. If patient is at all able, have him place brush as far back on tongue as he can without causing gagging, and brush forward. The patient stands this better if he uses the brush himself. This cleaning must not be omitted even if it is necessary for the nurse to use the brush.
   l. To wash the upper lingual surfaces, place the brush bristles up on the roof of the mouth and rotate the brush down over the gums and teeth surfaces. Continue until every surface is cleaned.
   m. To wash the lower lingual surfaces, place bristles on gums and rotate upward.

After-care of patient
1. Leave patient comfortable.

After-care of articles
1. Rinse the toothbrush and shake as much water as possible from it.
2. Replace in bag container or in bathroom.
3. Fold towel and hang on table.
4. Wash and boil kidney basin and mouthwash cup, dry, and replace in space provided.

References

Harmer, *Principles and Practice of Nursing*, pp. 108–11.
Lyon, "The Healthy Mouth," *American Journal of Nursing*, 1931, p. 1169.
Pickevill, *The Prevention of Dental Caries*, pp. 265–84.
Pyle, *Personal Hygiene*, pp. 17–26.

Special Care of the Mouth and Teeth

Purpose
1. To give adequate mouth care when patient is very ill.
2. To prevent formation of sordes.

Necessary articles
Tray.
Cotton pledgets, rolls, or sponges (few, as needed, on towel).
Curved forceps (Kelly).
Drinking tube.
Tongue blades.
Applicators, with cotton.
Lubricant (vaseline, cold cream, boric ointment, lanoline, or K. Y. Jelly).
Boric ointment, good treatment for dry, cracked lips and mucous membrane.
Mouthwash solution in cup.
Towel.
Paper bag.
Toothbrush.

Procedure
1. Proceed as in using brush except that the surfaces are first cleaned by sponging.
2. Moisten pledget and wash all surfaces thoroughly.
3. Then use brush to clean the teeth.
4. Use both pledget and brush on tongue with tongue extended.
5. Have patient rinse mouth by drawing some of the solution through the drinking tube or by raising the head and taking from the cup.
6. Rinse and have patient expectorate into basin.
7. Apply lubricant as follows:
   a. If mouth is parched and dry, some lubricant such as an albolene flavored with lemon juice is used. Pure cold cream or boric ointment can be used on the lips.
   b. Lemon juice and hydrogen peroxide, equal parts, is very good to soften sordes before washing and to keep mucous lining soft. Apply ointment to lips afterward.

Care of False Teeth

Procedure

1. Clean daily, and p. r. n.
2. When removed, place in a mouthwash cup of liquor antisepticus or boric acid solution.
3. *Should never be left on table, under pillow, or anywhere else where they might be broken or picked up with the soiled linen.*

References

Harmer, *Principles and Practice of Nursing,* p. 110.
Kelley, *Textbook of Nursing Technique,* pp. 40–41.

Care of the Hair *

THE TREATMENT FOR PEDICULOSIS CAPITAS AND FOR PEDICULOSIS CORPORIS

Purpose

1. To destroy pediculosis capitas.
2. To destroy pediculosis corporis.

General instructions

1. Avoid letting other patients know.
2. Do not allow patient up and around ward.
3. Cause patient as little embarrassment as possible.

Necessary articles

Tray.
Rubber pillowcase.
Tr. larkspur or tr. of staphisagria, 3 oz., or
Equal parts of olive oil and kerosene.
Triangular bandage.
Cotton balls in small basin.
Bath towel.

HEAD

Preparation of equipment

Prepare necessary articles and carry to bedside.

Preparation of patient

1. Screen completely, if in a ward; if in a room, place screen before door.
2. Arrange articles ready for use.

Procedure

1. Protect pillow with rubber pillowcase.
2. Cover pillow with bath towel placed lengthwise on pillow.
3. Using cotton balls, saturate hair and scalp thoroughly with prescribed solution. Have patient keep eyes closed.

* Moving pictures have been made of this procedure. See Preface, page iv.

4. Roll hair on top of patient's head.
5. Cover with triangular bandage and fasten snugly.
6. Leave this cap on from 12 to 24 hours.
7. Remove cap at end of this time and examine hair and scalp.
8. If nits are present, apply hot vinegar 105° F. in the same manner as prescribed solution.
9. Leave this cap on from 12 to 24 hours.
10. Remove and give shampoo.
11. Examine hair and scalp.
12. Repeat process if necessary.

After-care of equipment
1. Routine care of enamelware and rubber pillowcase.
2. Replace articles in space provided.

BODY

Procedure
1. Bathe daily with soap and water.
2. Follow by bath of bichloride of mercury solution 1/2000.
3. If ordered, mercury unguentin 33⅓ per cent, to be applied to hairy parts.
4. Hairy parts may be shaved, if necessary, with patient's permission.
5. Care of clothes:
   a. When undressing a patient with pediculosis corporis, spread a sheet on the floor and pile all clothing on this. Take care in handling clothes not to scatter the vermin to other beds. Hotbox or fumigate with sulphur all clothes that cannot be laundered. (Obtain permission of supervisor.)
   b. Put bed linen directly into bag used for isolation to be sent to laundry.

References
Harmer, *Principles and Practice of Nursing*, pp. 111–12.
Kelley, *Textbook of Nursing Technique*, p. 41.
Cavanagh, *Care of the Body*, pp. 145–57.

To Comb the Hair

Purpose
1. To stimulate the circulation.
2. To remove oil, dust, grime, etc.
3. To help prevent infection.

General instructions
1. Examine for pediculosis capitas or nits.
2. Avoid pulling.

3. Always wash comb after use on patient.
4. Comb hair every day after morning and evening care.
5. No patient is considered too ill to have her hair combed.

Procedure
1. Protect pillow with face towel.
2. Part hair in middle for two braids.
3. If tangled, wet with alcohol, separate into small sections, and comb, beginning at ends. Grasp the section being combed with the left hand and comb gently.
4. Braid in two braids in any way comfortable to patient, and fasten ends.
5. Occasionally it is necessary to cut matted hair. This cannot be done until head nurse secures *signed* statement from nearest relative granting permission to cut.

The Bed Shampoo *

Purpose
1. To wash the hair without discomfort to the patient and without getting the bed wet.
2. To stimulate the circulation.
3. To remove oil, dust, grime, etc.
4. To help prevent infection.

Necessary articles
Tray.
Rubber sheet, Kelly pad, or shampoo apron.
2 bath towels.
Washcloth.
Small pitcher of warm soap solution.
Newspaper to place on chair.
Rubber pillowcase.
2 pitchers of water, one 115° and the other 105° F.
Face towel.
Quart of water with 1 dram of vinegar if the water is hard. This is for the last rinse.
Foot tub or pail.

Preparation of equipment
1. Arrange small articles on tray and place tray on tub.
2. Carry all articles to bedside.

Preparation of patient
1. Move head of bed far enough out from wall so that bedside chair can be placed at head.†

---

* Moving pictures have been made of this procedure. See Preface, page iv.
† If it is not possible to pull head of bed from wall, patient can be moved to a diagonal position on bed and a chair placed at the side.

2. Put chair into position.
3. Place newspaper on chair.
4. Place tub or pail on chair.
5. Place tray with pitchers toward bed.
6. Move table up so that lower edge of table is even with head of bed.
7. Fanfold top bedding down to waist and replace with bath blanket.
8. Remove gown and place over foot of bed.
9. Remove pillows and place at foot of bed.

Procedure

1. Remove cotton pillowcase from one pillow; fold case and place over foot of bed.
2. Cover pillow with rubber pillowcase.
3. Cover pillow with bath towel placed lengthwise.
4. Place pillow under shoulders, with the upper edge even with shoulders.
5. Protect bed with rubber sheet, rolling sides to form a drainage pad, or use Kelly pad or shampoo apron, dropping free end between bars of bed and into tub or pail.
6. Loosen and comb patient's hair.
7. Moisten washcloth and cover patient's eyes.
8. Place face towel over head of bed.
9. Protecting the ears with right hand, pour water at a temperature of 105° over the hair. With tips of fingers use a circulatory movement over the scalp.
10. Pour soap into the hair and lather and rinse with clean warm water 3 times.
11. Squeeze water from hair.
12. Remove washcloth from eyes and place in pail or tub.
13. Remove Kelly pad and place in pail or tub.
14. Move patient back into position and place pillow covered with bath towel under head.
15. Dry the hair with bath towel over pillow.
16. When partially dry, place second bath towel under patient's head.
17. Spread hair out and dry.
18. Replace gown and remove bath blanket.
19. Replace table and chair.
20. Remove articles.
21. Comb the hair.
22. Remove rubber pillowcase on pillow and replace cotton pillowcase.
23. Leave bath towel over pillow if hair is slightly damp.

After-care of patient
1. Leave patient's bed, chair, and stand in correct position and in order.
2. Leave patient comfortable.

After-care of articles
1. Leave Kelly pad and washcloth in tub.
2. Place tray with other articles on tub.
3. Carry tray and tub to service room.
4. Wash and dry enamelware and replace in space provided.
5. Wash and dry Kelly pad and hang up to dry.
6. Place soiled linen in hamper.
7. Replace pillowcase in space provided.

Record
1. Hour.
2. Bed shampoo.
3. Effect on patient.

References
Harmer, *Principles and Practice of Nursing*, p. 112.
Kelley, *Textbook of Nursing Technique*, p. 41.

External Douche

Purpose
1. To cleanse external genitalia.
2. To aid in prevention of infection of perineal or rectal stitches.
3. To keep external genitalia dry and free from odor.

Necessary articles
Cart or tray covered with dressing towel containing:
Covered enamel can containing sterile cotton balls.
Covered enamel can containing sterile perineal pad.
Covered enamel instrument carrier containing sterile forceps or hemostats.
Sterile lifter in antiseptic solution.
Hemostat in antiseptic solution marked "contaminated."
Covered sterile pitcher containing sterile solution 105° F.
Folded newspaper or paper bag.
Kidney basin.
Can containing washed gauze (unsterile).

When given
1. Given routinely twice a day to abortion cases; all perineal repair patients; all patients with foul or profuse vaginal discharge; all patients with rectal operations.
2. Given following micturition and defecation in any of above conditions.

3. Given following micturition and defecation in all obstetrical cases.

Preparation of equipment
1. Fill sterile pitcher three-fourths full of sterile water 105° F. Take temperature with sterile solution thermometer.
2. Be sure there are instruments, cotton balls, pads, etc., on the tray before carrying it in.
3. Bring cart or tray to bedside; if tray, place on patient's bedside stand.
4. Warm bedpan and bring to bedside, place on chair.

Preparation of patient
1. Screen patient completely, if in a ward; if in a room, place screen before door.
2. Triangle bedcovers back; place paper bag or newspaper on foot of bed.
3. Remove pad with forceps from contaminated jar, place in paper bag.
4. Place patient on bedpan.

Procedure
1. After patient has used bedpan, fold back upper covers and drape thighs with sheet.
2. Remove cover from pitcher, hold pitcher in right hand 6 inches above patient, and pour water over parts.
3. Remove lid from can of cotton balls and hold with little finger of left hand.
4. With sterile lifters from antiseptic solution remove one forceps from instrument container; use in right hand.
5. Take cotton ball from can with sterile lifter; transfer to forceps in right hand.*
6. Cleanse and dry labia, using one downward stroke only for each cotton ball.
7. Discard cotton ball in paper bag with soiled pad. (Never place used cotton balls in bedpan.)
8. Use enough cotton balls to insure that labia are clean and dry.
9. Place used forceps in kidney basin and sterile forceps back into antiseptic solution.
10. Remove bedpan.
11. Remove perineal pad from can with sterile lifters and place on patient.
12. Turn patient on side and dry buttocks well.
13. If douche is given after defecation, it will be necessary to use

* Step 5 may be done as follows: Remove perineal pad from can, hold in right hand with sterile side up. Place on sterile pad 4 or 5 cotton balls from sterile can.

special care in cleaning stitches; this may have to be done while patient is on her side.

14. Pin pad in place and turn on back.
15. Remove paper bag and place on tray.

After-care of patient

1. Pull up covers and straighten bed.
2. Be sure that pad is kept in place.
3. Avoid letting patients handle soiled pads.

After-care of equipment

1. Care for bedpan in usual manner.
2. Discard newspaper and bag containing soiled cotton balls and pad.
3. Wash and boil used forceps for 10 minutes and replace in container.
4. Keep supply of cotton balls and pads replenished.

Record

1. In medication and treatment column: time, treatment.
2. In nurse's remarks column: any swelling or abnormal discharge.

References

Zabriskie, *Nurses' Handbook of Obstetrics*, pp. 301–02.
Reel, *Gynecology for Nurses*, pp. 176–77.
Kelley, *Textbook of Nursing Technique*, pp. 119–20.

V. CARDINAL SYMPTOMS AND OBSERVATIONS

Temperature, Pulse, and Respiration *

Purpose

1. To obtain objective criteria of the physical condition of the patient by comparison with normal conditions.
2. To aid in making a true diagnosis or prognosis in disease.

Temperature, pulse, and respiration are taken

1. B. i. d. on every patient in the hospital.
2. Q. 4 h., all patients with temperatures of 100° and above.
3. Any time ordered by attending physician or according to hospital routine.

Normal readings for adult

1. Temperature:
   a. Mouth — 98.6°.
   b. Rectal — 99.6°.
   c. Axillary — 97.6°.
2. Pulse: 72.
3. Respiration: 18.

MOUTH TEMPERATURE

General instructions

1. Do not take a temperature by mouth for 10 minutes after the patient has had something hot or cold to drink or eat.
2. Do not take temperature by mouth if patient is delirious, insane, uncooperative, or suffering from dyspnea.

Necessary articles

Tray.
Mouth thermometers; maximum number, 6.
5 containers:
   One, with layer of cotton on bottom, filled with bichloride of mercury 1/1000 with sodium oleate 0.2 per cent.
   One, with layer of cotton on bottom, filled with water.
   One, with layer of cotton on bottom, filled with soap solution.
   One for clean paper squares.
   One for soiled paper squares.
Pencil.
Temperature record.

Procedure

1. Place thermometers in container of bichloride solution and leave for 3 minutes.

* Moving pictures have been made of this procedure. See Preface, page iv

2. Carry tray to bedside of first patient.
3. Remove thermometer from bichloride and wipe with paper square.
4. Rinse in water and wipe with paper square.
5. Shake mercury to 95°.
6. Place end of thermometer containing the mercury under the tongue. See that the mouth is kept tightly closed.
7. Leave thermometer in the mouth for at least 3 minutes.
8. Count pulse for 1 minute by placing index and second finger over the radial artery at the wrist. Record on temperature record.
9. Count respiration for 1 minute before taking your fingers from the wrist. Record on temperature record.
10. Remove thermometer, read, and place in soap solution. Wipe with paper square. Replace in bichloride solution and leave for not less than 3 minutes. Record temperature on temperature record.

If there are several patients whose T. P. R. are being taken at this time the following procedure is used:

1. Repeat steps 3–6 three times.
2. Count pulse and respiration of third patient and record on temperature record.
3. Count pulse and respiration of second patient and record on temperature record.
4. Count pulse and respiration of first patient and record on temperature record.
5. Remove thermometer from first patient, wipe with paper square, read, and place in soap solution. Record temperature on temperature record.
6. Take tray with you and repeat step 5 for second and third patients.
7. Before placing 3 soiled thermometers in bichloride solution, remove clean thermometers preparatory to continuing with the next group of patients.

RECTAL TEMPERATURE

General instructions
1. Never allow patient to insert thermometer herself.
2. Never leave patient until thermometer has been removed.
3. Never take a rectal temperature if rectum has been operated on or is diseased.
4. An impacted rectum renders a rectal temperature inaccurate.

Necessary articles
Tray.
Rectal thermometer.

4 containers:
One, with layer of cotton on bottom, filled with bichloride of mercury 1/1000 with sodium oleate 0.2 per cent.
One, with layer of cotton on bottom, filled with soap solution.
One for clean paper squares.
One for soiled paper squares.
Tube or jar of vaseline.
Pencil.
Temperature record.

Procedure
1. Remove thermometer from bichloride solution.
2. Wipe with paper square.
3. Shake down to 96°.
4. Lubricate with vaseline.
5. Turn patient on side or leave on back if more convenient.
6. Insert thermometer slowly, bulb end first, up to 98°.
7. Allow to remain 5 minutes.
8. Take and record pulse and respiration.
9. Remove thermometer, wipe with paper square, and read.
10. Place in soap solution.
11. Remove from soap solution, wipe with paper square, and replace in bichloride solution and leave for 3 minutes.
12. Record temperature on temperature record.

Axillary Temperature

General instructions
1. Be sure that the axilla is dry.
2. Do not use too much friction in wiping away perspiration.

Necessary articles.
Same as for mouth.

Procedure
1. Use same technique for preparation of thermometer as for taking by mouth.
2. Remove sleeve of gown.
3. Place end of thermometer containing the mercury in the hollow of axilla.
4. Have patient hold arm down tightly with forearm across chest.
5. Leave for 10 minutes.
6. Remove and use the same technique as for mouth.

Care of tray
1. Empty containers, wash and refill after the b. i. d. temperatures and leave tray clean.

Record
1. Using scale of black figures at left side of chart, indicate temperature by a dot (pinhead size) in middle of space. Join preceding temperatures by a straight line. Use ruler.
2. Using scale of red figures at left side of chart, indicate pulse by a dot as for temperature. Join preceding pulse by a straight line. Use ruler.
3. Record respirations in column indicated.

References
Erdmann and Walsh, "Studies in Thermometer Technique," *Nursing Education Bulletin,* Vol. 2, No. 1, p. 18.
Harmer, *Principles and Practice of Nursing,* pp. 188–236.
Ashburn, "Bacteriological Study of Clinical Thermometer Technique," *American Journal of Nursing,* 1930, pp. 336–42.

Observation, Collection, and Care of Specimens

Purpose
1. To aid in diagnosing disease.
2. To aid in determining progress of disease.

General instructions
1. Secure proper receptacles for each kind of specimen.
2. Avoid contamination of specimen by having all receptacles clean.
3. Use no cracked receptacle.
4. Have quantity sufficient for examination.
5. Tubes containing liquid specimen should not be more than three-fourths full. (Avoid contamination of specimen from cork.)
6. Collect specimen at exact time ordered.
7. Be sure that label on specimen is clearly and completely made out.
8. Have sterile container if specimen is requested sterile or is for culture.
9. Explanation to patients about the saving of specimen (especially urine and feces) saves much delay in securing them.
10. Chart all specimens to laboratory.

Types of specimen ordered
1. Urine.
   a. Voided specimen:
      (1) Admissions: ordered routinely and collected by night nurse on following morning unless otherwise specified.
      (2) Pre-operative: whenever ordered.
      (3) Post-operative: whenever ordered.
      (4) Emergency or "stat" specimens.

(5) 24-hour specimen: hour closed determined by hospital.

(6) Special diagnostic tests: routine for each determined by each hospital:

    (a) Phenolsulphonephthalein (P. S. P.) test.

    (b) Dilution and concentration test.

    (c) Mosenthal test meal.

    (d) Glucose tolerance test.

  b. Catheterized specimens: any of the preceding may be requested obtained per catheter.

2. Feces:

  a. Transfer fecal material from bedpan to container with tongue blade and cover securely.

  b. Be sure that any unusual material, such as mucous, blood, etc., is included in specimen.

  c. Stool for amoeba should be sent to laboratory immediately in the bedpan, and given directly to technician. (After hours, place in incubator.)

  d. Stool for parasites or ova need not be warm, but should be soft or liquid.

  e. Stool for dysentery should be soft or liquid and should reach technician within 20 minutes after passage.

  f. Typhoid and dysentery stools handled with special technique in Communicable Disease Department.

3. Sputum:

  a. Instruct patient that a specimen is desired from the material expectorated from lungs or bronchi.

  b. Do not allow sputum to become contaminated outside of container. Cover securely.

  c. Special routine for handling in tuberculosis wards.

4. Stomach contents:

  a. Obtain by saving vomitus or remove contents by aspirating.

  b. Fractional expression:

    (1) Equipment is collected and prepared by nurse.

    (2) Tube is passed by doctor.

    (3) Gastric content is expressed by nurse.

    (4) Histamine, if ordered, given by nurse subcutaneously (average dose, 5 mg.).

5. Blood specimens:

  a. Wassermann: specimen should be taken to laboratory and placed in icebox immediately, or in accordance with routine of hospital.

  b. Chemistry: tube should contain a small amount of oxalate or some non-clotting agent (quantity about the size of a match head for 10 cc. blood).

  c. Sugar: tube contains oxalate.

d. Calcium: tube contains oxalate.
e. Culture: tube for culture *must* be sterile.
6. Body fluids:
   a. Types of body fluid:
      (1) Spinal.
      (2) Thoracic exudate.
      (3) Abdominal transudate.
   b. Tube for fluid must be sterile.
   c. Keep at room temperature; never in icebox.

Types of containers used
1. Urine:
   a. 4-oz. bottle: single specimen.
   b. Gallon bottle: 24-hour specimen.
   c. Special equipment for special tests.
2. Feces:
   Wax-lined pasteboard box.
3. Sputum:
   Small wax-lined pasteboard box.
4. Vomitus:
   Wax-lined pasteboard box, size according to amount.
5. Stomach contents:
   a. Entire contents: wax box.
   b. Fractional expression: glass test tubes.

Record
1. In treatment and medication column: time, type of specimen collected, purpose for which sent to laboratory, special comments, such as "catheterized," or other methods of collecting used, nurse's initials.

References
Kelley, *Textbook of Nursing Technique*, pp. 76–78.

Charting

Purpose
1. To form a part of the patient's complete clinical record.
2. To serve as an exact record of all treatments and medications given a patient during his hospital sojourn.
3. To give a picture of the patient's condition at all times while in the hospital.

General instructions
1. Charts are scientific documents, so the nurse's charting must be concise, accurate, and neat and must contain expert observations and explicit statements but omit nonessentials, unfamiliar technical terms, and diagnostic statements.

2. Charting must be so done as to be economical of time and space.
3. Charting is all printed in plain, easily legible, small characters.
4. Blot carefully after using ink. If a small mistake is made, the careful use of ink eradicator is allowed, but if many mistakes occur on a single page, the page must be copied; the original page must be retained in the chart, marked "copied" with the nurse's initials.
5. Each nurse does the charting for the patients assigned to her care and any other treatments she may carry out.
6. If in doubt about the spelling of a word, consult a dictionary.
7. The rule of silence should prevail at the chart desk; when charting, nurses should be as undisturbed as possible.
8. The heading of each page of chart must be completely filled out. Use patient's full name, with family name first: Smith, Caroline, not Mrs. F. C. Smith. Spell the name exactly as it appears on the admission card.

Procedure
1. Temperature sheet:
   a. Each day is headed with the month, day, and year in figures; for instance, 3/1/34.
   b. Day in hospital, day after operation, and hour filled in each day.
   c. Dots are made of uniform pinhead size. Join dots with a straight line, using a ruler.
   d. The temperature graph is made in black ink and the pulse graph in red ink.
   e. Record respirations in perpendicular figures in the column indicated.
   f. Stools are indicated by Roman numerals. Defecations are to be indicated for each patient at least once daily.
   g. Fluid totals are recorded by the night nurse at midnight in the spaces indicated.
2. Nurse's record:
   a. Diet is charted each day in the space indicated.
   b. Start each statement of observation at the column line. Indentation results in wasted space.
   c. Note the time of every observation or treatment charted. The nurse's initials follow all charting, including medications.
   d. Avoid repetition of unnecessary words or phrases, especially the word "patient." It is understood that all remarks refer to the patient unless otherwise indicated.
   e. To make charting consistent in regard to chemical symbols it would be necessary to use them throughout, which would

TEMPERATURE RECORD

Station_____Ward_____   DATE

NAME	4 A. M.			8 A. M.			12 N.			4 P. M.			8 P. M.			12 M.			DEF.
	T	P	R	T	P	R	T	P	R	T	P	R	T	P	R	T	P	R	

often mean long and complicated formulae; therefore avoid using them entirely.

f. Names of medications should be complete and never abbreviated. The following abbreviations may be used:

@, at
āā, of each
a. c., before meals
adm., admitted
ad lib., at pleasure

A. M., morning
amt., amount
ax., axilla (on temperature graph)
b. i. d., twice daily

c, with
C., centigrade
cc., cubic centimeter
en., enema (on temperature sheet)
F., Fahrenheit
gm., gram
gr., grain
gtt., drop
H., hour
(H), hypodermic
H. S., hours of sleep
m., minim
M., noon (meridian)
(M), mouth
mg., milligram
O. R., Operating Room
p. c., after meals
P. M., afternoon
p. r. n., as occasion requires

Pt., patient
q., every
q. i. d., four times a day
q. s., a sufficient quantity
(R) rectum (temperature graph)
℞, prescription
s̄, without
sig., give as follows
s. o. s., if necessary
spec., specimen
S. S., soap solution
ss, one-half
Sta., station
t. i. d., three times a day
trans., transferred
T. P. R., temperature, pulse, respiration
Wd., ward

g. A single red line is drawn across the chart at midnight to indicate the end of the day. The date of the next day is written in black ink on the first line below: e. g., 4/21/34.

h. Routine charting for patients not seriously ill includes a concise statement concerning condition of patient once during the day and a remark by night nurse indicating kind of night patient had. Morning care, evening care, and baths are charted when given.

i. Make statements concise and exact. Unless the definite weight or amount has been measured, use "approximately" or "about" so many cc. or gms. It is better to give approximate number of cc. than to use the term "small amount" or some other vague description.

j. The charting for each procedure is included in the directions for the procedure.

k. The patient's symptoms that are to be noted and charted are those the physician cannot himself discover. Statements should be definite. "Pain in the abdomen" is a worthless statement because of its indefiniteness and incompleteness. "A sharp intermittent pain in the right lower quadrant radiating toward the stomach" is one of value.

l. "Records are for all time, therefore make only significant and dignified entries; flippant, querulous, and unsubstantial entries are all unworthy of a mature worker."

Symptoms
  I. Objective
     A. Body discharges:
        a. Defecations:
           1. Unusual factors: mucus, gallstones, blood, tissue, un-
              digested food, parasites, clay-colored or tarry stools.
        b. Diaphoresis:
           1. Duration: greater part of A. M. or P. M., etc.
           2. Type: profuse, slight, moderate, local, general, cold,
              clammy.
        c. Emesis:
           1. Amount: in metric units if possible; otherwise large,
              small, moderate, scant.
           2. Duration: occasional, frequent, rare.
           3. Nature: projectile, without effort, followed by retch-
              ing, forcible, unrestrained.
           4. Characteristics: green, yellow, blood-tinged, hemate-
              mesis (blood), coffee grounds, bile, containing mu-
              cus, appearance of medicine.
           5. Unusual features: cardiac or respiratory difficulty,
              odor of feces, undigested food, etc.
        d. Excretions:
           1. Source: nasal, aural, oral, vaginal, rectal, or urethral
              sources, surgical wounds.
           2. Nature: watery, lacremal, sanguineous, sero-puru-
              lent, purulent, mucus.
           3. Amount: slight, moderate, profuse, scant.
           4. Odor: none, slight, foul.
        e. Expectoration:
           1. Nature: tenacious, liquid, mucus, purulent, blood-
              tinged, foul odor, hemoptysis (blood-spitting).
           2. Amount: scant, rare, profuse, moderate, occasional.
     B. Convulsions:
        1. Duration of attack.
        2. Type: tonic (continuous); clonic (intermittent).
        3. Area of body involved: local (spasms), general (epilep-
           tiform), tetanic, hysteric, eclamptic.
        4. Changes in pulse or respiration.
        5. Color or expression.
     C. Cough:
        1. Duration: continuous, spasmodic, occasional, rare.
        2. Type: vigorous, weak, rasping, strong, hoarse, whoop-
           ing, productive, nonproductive, etc.
        3. Effects on patient: tiring, exhaustive, with effort, with
           ease.

D. Cyanosis:
1. Area involved: lips, fingertips, face, nose.
2. Severity and increase of: slight, deep, definite, temporary, permanent.
E. Eyes:
1. Appearance: sunken, protruding, glazed, dull, bloodshot, jaundiced.
2. Eyeballs: rolling, twitching, motionless, fixed.
3. Photophobia: sensitivity to light.
4. Pupils: dilated as in real pain or from fright, unequal dilation, contracted pin point.
F. Facial observations:
1. Color: pallor, flushed, cyanotic, hectic flush, livid.
2. Muscular contractions: twitchings at corner of lips, nose, etc.
3. Swelling or edema around eyes or lips.
4. Deformities.
5. Expression: anxious, indifferent, dull, worried, alert, evincing pain, pallor about lips, depressed, responsive.
G. Hands:
1. Condition: cold, warm, hot, dry, moist, emaciated, clammy.
2. Movements: inactive, inaccurate, listless, restless, picks at bed clothing, tremulous, firm.
H. Joints:
1. Unusual factors: grating, stiffness, swollen, tender, pain accompanying motion, deformities, distorted, enlarged.
I. Mental characteristics:
1. Conditions: active, anxious, apathetic, depressed, dull, elated, irritable, nervous, phlegmatic, melancholic, wandering in speech and ideas, sluggish, talkative, confused, hypersensitive, etc.
2. Consciousness: Partial (semi-conscious), stuporous, entirely lacking.
3. Delirium: low muttering, noisy, screaming, constant, occasional.
4. Irrational: hallucinations of sight, sound, or odor; attempting to get out of bed; disoriented as to time, place, etc.
J. Mouth:
1. Breath: fetid from disease, feverish; heavy; hot; foul from decayed teeth; sour; sweetish; bears odor of alcohol, acetone, urine, drugs, etc.
2. Gums: grayish or with blue line along margin, bleeding, receding, swollen, red.

3. Lips: blue, dry, cracked, pale, cherry red.

4. Tongue: black streaked, cherry red, coated all over, coated with margins, bright red, brown, grayish white, yellow, dry, furred, ulcerated, enlarged, swollen, tremulous.

K. Movement of body:

    1. Nature: restless, twitching, turning from side to side.

L. Skin:

    1. Color: flushed, diffuse or localized; pallor, sudden, transient, progressive; bluish tinge; grayish; cyanosed; livid, jaundiced.

    2. Nature: dry, cracked, hot, warm, feverish, cold, clammy, sensitive to heat or cold, itching.

    3. Unusual conditions: Erythema, pin point, spotted; urticara, eczema, petechia, purpura, papules, maculae, vesicles.

M. Sleep:

    1. Duration: continuous, at intervals (specify time).

    2. Character: normal, quiet, restful, light, disturbed (state type of restlessness — for instance, moans in sleep, is easily awakened — and methods used to control), insomnia.

N. Syncope:

    1. Objective symptoms: small, weak pulse, shallow respirations; unconscious, prostrate on ground.

    2. Methods used to relieve.

O. Tympanites:

    1. Character: slight, moderate, pronounced.

    2. Methods used to reduce.

    3. Results secured.

P. Weight:

    1. Unusual conditions: obese, malnourished, emaciated, skin loose, marked distribution of adipose tissue.

II. Subjective:

    1. Nature: loss of appetite, condition of appetite; burning sensations; fear of darkness, being alone, etc.; deafness; dizziness; hot and cold flashes; headache; hunger; itching; nausea; numbness; pain; pressure; thirst; throbbing sensation; tingling sensation; touch and visual disturbances.

    2. Location, if possible.

    3. Cause, if possible.

    4. Duration, if possible.

    5. Methods used to relieve.

    6. Effects of methods employed.

After-care of chart

1. When patient is dismissed, the chart is checked to make sure that all pages are completely headed. It is arranged in the proper order and after going through the discharge routine of the hospital is filed in the Record Room for future reference and study.

2. Graduate nurses on duty in a private home should keep as complete and exact a chart as would be kept in a hospital. Printed chart forms are available in hospital supply houses at a nominal cost. The chart should be offered to the doctor at the conclusion of the case; if he does not care for it, it is usually destroyed.

References

Ewing, "Achievement in the Form of Charting," *American Journal of Nursing*, 1931, p. 554.

———, "Introduction to Clinical Charting," *American Journal of Nursing*, 1931, p. 169.

Basche, "Concerning Charting," *American Journal of Nursing*, 1928, p. 17.

Harmer, *Principles and Practice of Nursing*, pp. 58–70.

Positions and Draping for Examinations and Treatments

Purpose

1. To protect the patient during examination and treatment.

2. For the comfort of the patient while different parts of the body are being examined.

General instructions

1. Avoid all unnecessary exposure of the body.

2. In a ward protect the patient from other patients by the use of screens.

3. Drape so that the outline of the patient's figure will not be discernible.

4. Keep patient covered until the physician comes.

5. Tell patient the reason for the examination.

6. If a complete physical examination is to be made, replace the covers with a bath blanket.

7. Have all the necessary articles at hand.

8. See that the windows are closed and that the shades are up.

Necessary articles

1. Physical examinations:

Tray.	Flashlight.
Wooden tongue depressors.	Red and blue pencils.
Paper bag.	Tape measure.
Face towel.	Safety pins.

Doctor's towels.   Tuning fork.
Applicator with pin.   Glass slides.
Percussion hammer.

Note. — If examination of eye, ear, and throat is to be made, additional articles must be provided.

2. Gynecological examination:
   Tray.   Glove powder.
   Large sheet.   Doctor's towels.
   Sterile gloves.   Lubricant.
   Sterile perineal pad.   Rubber protector.
   Paper bag.   Bedpan cover.

Positions
1. Dorsal:
   a. Patient flat on back, one pillow under his head.
   b. Knees separated and slightly flexed.
2. Knee-chest:
   a. Allow one small pillow for head.
   b. Patient rests on chest and knees; knees slightly separated; face turned on side resting on the pillow; thighs perpendicular; arms free at both sides.
3. Sims:
   a. Patient lies on left side; right knee flexed and drawn up nearly to abdomen; left knee slightly flexed; left arm drawn under the side to back; right arm free in front.
4. Lithotomy:
   a. In bed: patient on back across bed, buttocks slightly beyond edge of mattress, hips slightly elevated with pillows; knees flexed on abdomen and held in position by strap or folded sheet passed upward over one shoulder, back of the neck, and down over opposite shoulder, and pinned about flexed knees.
   b. On examining table: patient in dorsal position with knees flexed. The feet are placed in stirrups at foot of table.
5. Trendelenburg:
   a. Patient lies on back on examining table, thighs and trunk elevated on an inclined plane of 45 degrees. Legs bent at knees down on other side of plane.
   b. Shoulder supports are used to prevent patient from slipping.

Types of examinations
1. Throat:
   a. Have patient in position so that a strong light, at the examiner's back, can be thrown upon throat of patient.

b. If examiner uses head mirror, have light always in front, either natural or artificial.

c. Always hold tongue depressor in the middle so that the fingers do not touch the portion that is to go into patient's mouth.

d. After a tongue blade has been used, it should never be placed on a chair, bed, or table. Put immediately in a paper bag or emesis basin, and into the garbage can as soon as possible.

2. Chest:

a. Up patient:

(1) Remove all clothing from upper part of body.

(2) Place sheet folded diagonally about shoulders, pinning it in front.

(3) Have patient sit on stool or chair so that front and back are accessible.

(4) When doctor examines front of chest, fold the sheet back over shoulders; when the back of chest, turn the sheet around with the opening in the back. Then fold back over the shoulders.

b. Bed patient:

(1) Remove all but 1 pillow.

(2) Always hold towel between patient's face and doctor's head.

(3) If patient is able to sit up in bed, drape as for up patient.

(4) If unable to sit up, either remove gown and place a towel over anterior chest, or roll up hem of gown so that it does not interfere with examination.

(5) To examine back, turn patient on his side away from doctor and drape as for anterior chest, or have patient sit up in bed. Support lower back with pillow. Place towel over posterior chest, and gown over anterior chest.

3. Abdomen:

a. Have patient lie in dorsal position with knees flexed to relax abdominal muscles.

b. Turn all bedding back to pubes and groins and cover patient with towel or blanket.

c. Place towel over abdomen and at the same time draw up patient's gown and roll it just above waistline.

d. During examination the towel is removed from abdomen and placed over the pubes.

4. Lower extremities:

a. Loosen bedding from foot of bed.

b. Fold spread and blanket upward.

c. Leave sheet to prevent unnecessary exposure of extremities.

d. When both legs are being examined, bring sheet between the thighs.

5. Rectal:
   a. Screen patient.
   b. Fanfold upper bedding to foot of bed and at the same time cover patient with an extra sheet.
   c. Place patient in dorsal, knee-chest, or Sims position, usually dorsal with knees flexed.
   d. Use sheet diagonally and wrap both feet and legs in each corner.
   e. Or have patient flex the knee on the side on which the doctor stands, and turn back corner covers. Put a rubber protector and a bedpan cover under the buttocks.
   f. Open package of gloves and hold right glove for the doctor to put on. Uncover lubricant.
   g. Turn back corner of sheet between knees.

6. Vaginal:
   a. Have external parts scrupulously clean.
   b. Have patient void.
   c. Have patient relax as much as possible by taking a series of long, deep breaths.
   d. Fanfold the bedding and drape patient with sheet folded diagonally as for rectal examination.
   e. Assist doctor with glove and lubricant.
   f. Protect patient's modesty and sensibilities by control of speech and facial expression.

After-care of equipment
1. Leave tray clean and equipped for future use.
2. Wash gloves with cold water, then with soap and warm water, and boil 3 minutes. Dry thoroughly on both sides.

Record
1. Hour of examination.
2. By whom performed.

References
Harmer, *Principles and Practice of Nursing*, pp. 607–13.
Young, *Textbook of Gynecology*, pp. 44–50.
Reed, *Gynecology for Nurses*, pp. 106–13.

VI. ENEMATA AND RECTAL FEEDINGS

General instructions
1. Do not expose patient unnecessarily.
2. Protect bed from excretions and odor.
3. Lubricate tip and insert slowly and gently.
4. The presence of air in the tubing retards the flow of the solution, so the air should be removed by allowing some solution to flow through the tube before it is inserted. This also warms the tubing so that it causes less discomfort when inserted.
5. Allow solution to flow at rate of approximately 1 quart in 8 minutes.
6. Position of patient:
   a. Preferably on left side with knees flexed, right more than left.
   b. Dorsal recumbent if movement is difficult for patient.

Cleansing or Evacuating Enema

Purposes
1. To soften feces.
2. To stimulate peristalsis by distending the colon and rectum.
3. To cause a free evacuation.

Solutions used
1. Soap solution.
2. Normal saline solution.
3. Tap water.

Temperature of solution
1. 100° to 105° F.

Amount
1. Child or small adult, 2–3 pints.
2. Normal or large adult, 3–4 pints.

Necessary articles
Irrigating can, with 3 feet of rubber tubing and stopcock and glass connector on end. Rectal tip or rectal tube, size 22 or 30, in kidney basin, vaseline, and square of toilet paper for applying.
Wooden block 16 inches high for holding can.
Bedpan and toilet paper.
Bath blanket.
Rubber protector covered with clean bedpan cover.
Tray.

Preparation of equipment
1. Close stopcock on tubing of irrigating can and prepare solution in can by dissolving pure white toilet soap (Ivory) in hot water.
2. Dilute to the proper amount and correct temperature. Test with bath thermometer.
   Skim off suds with hand.
3. Put vaseline on square of toilet paper and lubricate end of rectal tube for 4 inches. Place in kidney basin.
4. Cover tray with bedpan cover.
5. Carry tray placed on bedpan to bedside.
6. Place bedpan on chair and tray on bedside stand.

Preparation of patient
1. Tell patient what the treatment is to be.
2. Screen completely, if in a ward; if in a room, place screen before door.
3. Fanfold top bedding down and replace with bath blanket.
4. Fold gown up over chest.
5. Place covered rubber protector under hips.
6. Turn patient on left side if possible, with knees flexed, right more than left; if patient prefers, dorsal recumbent position is satisfactory.

Procedure
1. Place can block on stand, and irrigating can on block.
2. Attach rectal tube to rubber tubing.
3. Open stopcock and expel air from tubing.
4. Insert tube gently for about 2 inches, open stopcock and allow fluid to enter rectum for 1 minute, then insert tube 2 inches more.
5. Regulate flow according to patient's ability to retain solution.
6. When solution has been taken, close stopcock, withdraw rectal tube, disconnect from rubber tubing, wrap toilet paper around it, and place in kidney basin.
7. Instruct patient to retain solution from 5 to 10 minutes if possible.
8. Place irrigating can on tray. Cover tray.
9. Place patient on bedpan or put within easy reach. Also place signal light and toilet paper so as to be accessible.
10. Carry tray and block to service room.
11. Leave patient alone for 15 minutes or until she calls.

After-care of patient
1. Remove bedpan, cover, carry to service room, note contents, and clean in the usual way.
2. Bring basin of water to bedside.

3. Wash patient's hands.
4. Turn on side, cleanse and dry parts thoroughly.
5. Remove rubber protector and cover.
6. Straighten gown, pull up covers, and remove bath blanket. If bath blanket is not soiled, fold and place in space provided; otherwise carry out with rest of material and put with soiled linen.
7. Open window and remove screen.
8. Note appearance of patient.
9. Carry out basin of water and rubber protector.

After-care of equipment
1. Rinse irrigating can and tubing with warm water. Leave stopcock open.
2. Force cold water through rectal tube. Be sure that all fecal matter is removed. If necessary, use applicator. Wash with soap and warm water in kidney basin.
3. Wash kidney basin.
4. Place irrigating can and tubing, kidney basin, and enema tube in sterilizer. Boil 3 minutes.
5. Remove from sterilizer, rinse rubber material in cold water, and dry.
6. Replace all equipment on clean tray, cover, and replace on shelf.
7. Wash, dry, and replace basin.
8. Wash and dry rubber protector, cover with clean cover, and replace on tray.
9. Wash and dry hands.

Record
1. Check and write time of giving in red in left-hand margin opposite order in doctor's order book.
2. In treatment and medication column: the time, kind of solution, character, and amount of results, and by whom given (initials). In nurse's remarks column: general effect of treatment.
3. Indicate with "En." in stool space on temperature sheet.

References
Harmer, *Principles and Practice of Nursing*, pp. 160–64.
Kelley, *Textbook of Nursing Technique*, pp. 78–84.
Greisheimer, *Physiology and Anatomy*, pp. 391–93.

Carminative Enema

Purpose
1. To relieve distention caused by flatus.

Solutions usually ordered
1. Turpentine, 1 dram; olive oil, 4 ounces.
2. Noble's enema: turpentine, 1 dram; glycerine, 2 ounces; magnesium sulphate, 3 ounces; water, 4 ounces.
3. Tr. asafetida, 2 drams; water, 4–6 ounces.
4. Milk, 8 ounces; molasses, 8 ounces.

Temperature of solution
1. 100°–105° F.

Necessary articles
Funnel with rectal tube, size 23, in kidney basin.
Vaseline and square of toilet paper for applying.
Small rubber protector.
4 bedpan covers.
Bath blanket.
Graduate with solution ordered.
Bedpan and toilet paper.
Tray.

Preparation of equipment
1. Prepare solution ordered at the correct temperature. Test with bath thermometer.
2. Put vaseline on square of toilet paper and lubricate end of rectal tube for 4 inches.
3. Attach rectal tube to funnel. Place in kidney basin.
4. Cover tray with bedpan cover.
5. Place all articles on tray and cover with bedpan cover.
6. Carry tray placed on bedpan to bedside.
7. Place bedpan on chair and tray on bedside stand.

Preparation of patient
1. Tell patient what the treatment is to be.
2. Screen completely, if in a ward; if in a room, place screen before door.
3. Fanfold top bedding down and replace with bath blanket.
4. Fold gown up over chest.
5. Place covered rubber protector under hips.
6. Turn patient on left side if possible, with knees flexed, right more than left; if patient prefers, dorsal recumbent position is satisfactory.

Procedure
1. Pour a small quantity of solution into funnel, enough to expel air from tubing.
2. Insert tube gently for about 2 inches.
3. Pour in about ½ ounce of solution, then insert tube 2 inches more.

4. Regulate flow according to patient's ability to retain solution.
5. When solution has been taken, clamp tube with fingers and withdraw.
6. Wrap toilet paper around tube and place in kidney basin.
7. Instruct patient to retain solution 5 to 10 minutes if possible.
8. Cover tray.
9. Place patient on bedpan or put within easy reach of patient. Also place signal light and toilet paper so as to be accessible.
10. Carry tray to service room.
11. Leave patient alone for 15 minutes or until she calls.

After-care of patient
1. Remove bedpan, cover, carry to service room, note contents, and clean in the usual way.
2. Bring basin of water to bedside.
3. Wash patient's hands.
4. Turn on side, cleanse and dry parts thoroughly.
5. Remove rubber protector and cover.
6. Straighten gown, pull up covers, and remove bath blanket. If bath blanket is not soiled, fold and place in space provided; otherwise carry out with rest of material and put with soiled linen.
7. Open window and remove screen.
8. Note appearance of patient.
9. Carry out basin of water and rubber protector.

After-care of equipment
1. Force cold water through rectal tube. Be sure that all fecal matter is removed. If necessary, use applicator. Wash with soap and warm water in kidney basin.
2. Wash kidney basin, funnel, and graduate.
3. Place rectal tube in kidney basin and graduate in sterilizer.
4. Boil for 3 minutes.
5. Remove from sterilizer, rinse rubber material in cold water, and dry. Dry funnel, kidney basin, and graduate.
6. Replace articles in space provided.
7. Wash and dry rubber protector.
8. Wash and dry hands.

Record
1. In treatment and medication column: time, name of solution, amount, temperature, results, i. e., amount of flatus and feces expelled.
2. In nurse's remarks column: pain caused by treatment, relief obtained, or any other observation made.
3. Initial recording.

References

Harmer, *Principles and Practice of Nursing,* pp. 163–64.

Kelley, *Textbook of Nursing Technique,* pp. 84–86.

Emollient, Sedative, and Stimulating Enemata

Purpose

1. Emollient: to soothe the irritated mucous membranes.
2. Sedative: to quiet the patient.
3. Stimulating: to stimulate in cases of shock or collapse.

General instructions

1. Keep patient quiet after giving the enema.
2. Avoid all stimuli, either mental or physical, that might excite peristalsis.
3. Have rectum and colon free from feces.

Solutions usually ordered

1. Emollient:
   a. Cornstarch, 1 dram; cold water, 1½ ounces. Mix to a smooth paste and add 5 ounces of boiling water. Boil one or two minutes and cool to 105° F. If laudanum or opium is prescribed, add to the enema just before giving.
   b. Flaxseed, 33 cc.; cold water, 1 pint. Boil for 10 minutes, strain, and inject while warm.
2. Sedative:
   a. Chloral hydrate. Sodium bromide. Paraldehyde. Mix medication ordered with 6 ounces of water.
3. Stimulating:
   a. Strong black coffee, 5–6 ounces.

Temperature of solution

1. 100°–105° F.

Necessary articles

Funnel with rectal tube, size 22, in kidney basin.

Vaseline and square of toilet paper for applying.

Small rubber protector.

3 bedpan covers.

Bath blanket.

Graduate with solution ordered.

Tray.

Preparation of equipment

1. Prepare solution ordered at correct temperature. Test with bath thermometer.
2. Put vaseline on square of toilet paper and lubricate end of rectal tube for 4 inches.
3. Attach rectal tube to funnel. Place in kidney basin.

4. Cover tray with bedpan cover.
5. Place all articles on tray and cover with bedpan cover.
6. Carry tray to bedside and place on bedside stand.

Preparation of patient
1. Tell patient what the treatment is to be.
2. Screen completely, if in a ward; if in a room, place screen before door.
3. Fanfold top bedding down and replace with bath blanket.
4. Fold gown up over chest.
5. Place covered rubber protector under hips.
6. Turn patient on left side, if possible, with knees flexed, right more than left; if patient prefers, dorsal recumbent position is satisfactory.

Procedure
1. Pour small quantity of solution into funnel, enough to expel air from tubing.
2. Insert tube gently for about 2 inches.
3. Pour in about ½ ounce of solution, then insert tube 2 inches more.
4. Regulate flow according to patient's ability to retain solution.
5. When solution has been taken, clamp tube with fingers and withdraw.
6. Wrap toilet paper around tube and place in kidney basin.
7. Instruct patient to retain solution. This type of enema is usually retained for several hours.
8. Cover tray and remove to service room.

After-care of patient
1. Leave rubber protector and cover under patient.
2. Straighten gown, pull up covers, and remove bath blanket. If bath blanket is not soiled, fold and place in space provided; otherwise carry out with rest of material and put with soiled linen.
3. Remove screen and leave patient comfortable and unit in order.

After-care of equipment
1. Force cold water through rectal tube. Be sure that all fecal matter is removed. If necessary, use applicators. Wash with soap and water in kidney basin.
2. Wash funnel, kidney basin, and graduate.
3. Place rectal tube, kidney basin, funnel, and graduate in sterilizer. Boil 3 minutes.
4. Remove from sterilizer, rinse rectal tube in cold water and dry. Dry funnel, kidney basin, and graduate.

5. Replace articles in space provided.
6. Wash and dry hands.

Record
1. In medication and treatment column: time, kind, strength, amount of solution, retention.
2. In nurse's remarks column: general effects obtained, if observable.
3. All charting is followed by the nurse's initials.

References
Harmer, *Principles and Practice of Nursing*, pp. 165–69.
Kelley, *Textbook of Nursing Technique*, pp. 86–88.

Medicated Enemata

Purpose
1. Anthelmintic: to destroy worms.
2. Antiseptic: to destroy bacteria.
3. Astringent: to contract the tissues and blood vessels.
4. Cathartic: to prevent the absorption of water, thus causing distention of the intestines and stimulating evacuation.

Solutions usually ordered
1. Anthelmintic:
    a. Infusion of quassia, 6 ounces, prepared by pouring 1 pint of water over 1 ounce of quassia chips and straining the water off when cold.
    b. Tannic acid, prepared by pouring 1 pint of hot water over 30 grains of the acid. Cool to correct temperature.
    c. Alum, prepared by pouring 1 pint of hot water over 30 grains of the drug. Cool to correct temperature.
2. Antiseptic:
    a. Silver nitrate, 10 grains; water, 1 pint.
3. Astringent:
    a. Alum.
    b. Tannic acid.

Temperature of solution
1. 100°–105° F.

Necessary articles
Funnel with rectal tube, size 23, in kidney basin.
Vaseline and square of toilet paper for applying.
Small rubber protector.
4 bedpan covers.
Bath blanket.
Graduate with solution ordered.
Bedpan and toilet paper.
Tray.

Preparation of equipment

1. Prepare solution ordered at the correct temperature. Test with bath thermometer.
2. Put vaseline on square of toilet paper and lubricate end of rectal tube for 4 inches.
3. Attach rectal tube to funnel. Place in kidney basin.
4. Cover tray with bedpan cover.
5. Place all articles on tray and cover with bedpan cover.
6. Carry tray placed on bedpan to bedside.
7. Place bedpan on chair and tray on bedside stand.

Preparation of patient

1. Tell patient what the treatment is to be.
2. Screen completely, if in a ward; if in a room, place screen before door.
3. Fanfold top bedding down and replace with bath blanket.
4. Fold gown up over chest.
5. Place covered rubber protector under hips.
6. Turn patient on left side if possible, with knees flexed, right more than left; if patient prefers, dorsal recumbent position is satisfactory.

Procedure

1. Pour a small quantity of solution into funnel, enough to expel air from tubing.
2. Insert tube gently for about 2 inches.
3. Pour in about ½ ounce of solution, then insert tube 2 inches more.
4. Regulate flow according to patient's ability to retain solution.
5. When solution has been taken, clamp tube with fingers and withdraw.
6. Wrap toilet paper around tube and place in kidney basin.
7. Instruct patient to retain solution 15 to 30 minutes, if possible.
8. Cover tray.
9. Place patient on bedpan or put within easy reach of patient. Also place signal light and toilet paper so as to be accessible.
10. Carry tray to service room.
11. Leave patient alone for 15 minutes or until she calls.

After-care of patient

1. Remove bedpan, cover, carry to service room, note contents, and clean in the usual way.
2. Bring basin of water to bedside.
3. Wash patient's hands.
4. Turn on side, cleanse and dry parts thoroughly.
5. Remove rubber protector and cover.
6. Straighten gown, pull up covers, and remove bath blanket. If

bath blanket is not soiled, fold and place in space provided; otherwise carry out with rest of material and put with soiled linen.
7. Open window and remove screen.
8. Note appearance of patient.
9. Carry out basin of water and rubber protector.

After-care of equipment
1. Force cold water through rectal tube. Be sure that all fecal matter is removed. If necessary, use applicator. Wash with soap and warm water in kidney basin.
2. Wash kidney basin, funnel, and graduate.
3. Place rectal tube, kidney basin, and graduate in sterilizer. Boil 3 minutes.
4. Remove from sterilizer, rinse rubber material in cold water, and dry. Dry funnel, kidney basin, and graduate.
5. Replace articles in space provided.
6. Wash and dry rubber protector.
7. Wash and dry hands.

Record
1. In medication and treatment column: time, name, amount, strength and temperature of solution, length of retention, results as to defecation, etc.
2. In nurse's remarks column: systemic effects, if observable.
3. All charting is followed by nurse's initials.

References
Harmer, *Principles and Practice of Nursing*, p. 162.
Kelley, *Textbook of Nursing Technique*, pp. 89–90.

Nutritive Enema

Purpose
1. To provide nourishment.

General instructions
1. Utmost patience and skill should be used to secure the best possible results.
2. Patient must be free from all causes of mental excitement and of physical discomforts and unrest.
3. The condition of the bowel must be clean and healthy.
4. Foods must be predigested.
5. Small amounts only should be given (4–8 ounces every 4–6 hours.)
6. Injections should be given slowly.
7. After injection, the patient should be kept as quiet and comfortable as possible.

Necessary articles
Funnel with rectal tube, size 22, in kidney basin.
Vaseline and square of toilet paper for applying.
Small rubber protector.
3 bedpan covers.
Bath blanket.
Graduate with solution ordered.
Tray.

Preparation of equipment
1. Prepare solution ordered at correct temperature. Test with bath thermometer.
2. Put vaseline on square of toilet paper and lubricate end of rectal tube for 4 inches.
3. Attach rectal tube to funnel. Place in kidney basin.
4. Cover tray with bedpan cover.
5. Place all articles on tray and cover with bedpan cover.
6. Carry tray to bedside and place on bedside stand.

Preparation of patient
1. Tell patient what the treatment is to be.
2. Screen completely, if in ward; if in room, place screen before door.
3. Fanfold top bedding down and replace with bath blanket.
4. Fold gown up over chest.
5. Place covered rubber protector under hips.
6. Turn patient on left side, if possible, with knees flexed, right more than left; if patient prefers, dorsal recumbent position is satisfactory.

Procedure
1. Pour a small quantity of solution into funnel, enough to expel air from tubing.
2. Insert tube gently for about 2 inches.
3. Pour in about ½ ounce of solution, then insert tube 2 inches more.
4. Regulate flow according to patient's ability to retain solution.
5. When solution has been taken, clamp tube with fingers and withdraw.
6. Wrap toilet paper around tube and place in kidney basin.
7. Instruct patient to retain solution.

After-care of patient
1. Leave rubber protector and cover under the patient.
2. Straighten gown, pull up covers, and remove bath blanket. If bath blanket is not soiled, fold and place in space provided; otherwise carry out with rest of material and put with soiled linen.

3. Remove screen and leave patient comfortable and unit in order.

After-care of equipment
1. Force cold water through rectal tube. Be sure that all fecal matter is removed. If necessary, use applicator. Wash with soap and water in kidney basin.
2. Wash funnel, kidney basin, and graduate.
3. Place rectal tube, kidney basin, funnel, and graduate in sterilizer. Boil 3 minutes.
4. Remove from sterilizer, rinse rectal tube in cold water and dry. Dry funnel, kidney basin, and graduate.
5. Replace articles in space provided.
6. Wash and dry hands.

Oil Enema

Purpose
1. To aid in softening feces.
2. To act as an emollient to the irritated mucosa of the intestines.

Solutions usually ordered
1. Olive oil, 6 ounces.
2. Castor oil and glycerine, 2 ounces each.

Temperature of solution
1. 100°–105° F.

Necessary articles
Funnel with rectal tube, size 22, in kidney basin.
Vaseline and square of toilet paper for applying.
Small rubber protector.
3 bedpan covers.
Bath blanket.
Graduate with solution ordered.
Tray.

Preparation of equipment
1. Prepare solution ordered at correct temperature. Test with bath thermometer.
2. Put vaseline on square of toilet paper and lubricate end of rectal tube for 4 inches.
3. Attach rectal tube to funnel. Place in kidney basin.
4. Cover tray with bedpan cover.
5. Place all articles on tray and cover with bedpan cover.
6. Carry tray to bedside and place on bedside stand.

Preparation of patient
1. Tell patient what the treatment is to be.

2. Screen completely, if in a ward; if in room, place screen before door.
3. Fanfold top bedding down and replace with bath blanket.
4. Fold gown up over chest.
5. Place covered rubber protector under hips.
6. Turn patient on left side, if possible, with knees flexed, right more than left; if patient prefers, dorsal recumbent position is satisfactory.

Procedure
1. Pour small quantity of solution into funnel, enough to expel air from tubing.
2. Insert tube gently for about 2 inches.
3. Pour in about ½ ounce of solution, then insert tube 2 inches more.
4. Regulate flow according to patient's ability to retain solution.
5. When solution has been taken, clamp tube with fingers and withdraw.
6. Wrap toilet paper around tube and place in kidney basin.
7. Instruct patient to retain solution. This type of enema is usually retained for several hours and is then followed by a soap-suds enema.
8. Cover tray and remove to service room.

After-care of patient
1. Leave rubber protector and cover under patient.
2. Straighten gown, pull up covers, and remove bath blanket. If bath blanket is not soiled, fold and place in space provided; otherwise carry out with rest of material and put with soiled linen.
3. Remove screen and leave patient comfortable and unit in order.

After-care of equipment
1. Force cold water through rectal tube. Be sure that all fecal matter is removed. If necessary, use applicator. Wash with soap and water in kidney basin.
2. Wash funnel, kidney basin, and graduate.
3. Place rectal tube, kidney basin, funnel, and graduate in sterilizer. Boil 3 minutes.
4. Remove from sterilizer, rinse rectal tube in cold water and dry. Dry funnel, kidney basin, and graduate.
5. Replace articles in space provided.
6. Wash and dry hands.

Record
1. In medication and treatment column: time, kind, amount, and retention of oil.

2. In nurse's remarks column: general effects, comfort or discomfort.

3. All charting is followed by nurse's initials.

References
Harmer, *Principles and Practice of Nursing*, p. 162.
Kelley, *Textbook of Nursing Technique*, pp. 88–89.

Proctoclysis

Purpose
1. To supply the body with fluid.

Necessary articles
Bath blanket.
Standard.
Irrigating can and double tubing.
Rectal tube or catheter, size Fr. 18, 10, Am. 12.
Vaseline and paper square for applying.
Narrow adhesive strip for securing tube if patient is restless.
Bedpan cover.
Rubber protector.
Kidney basin.
Tray.

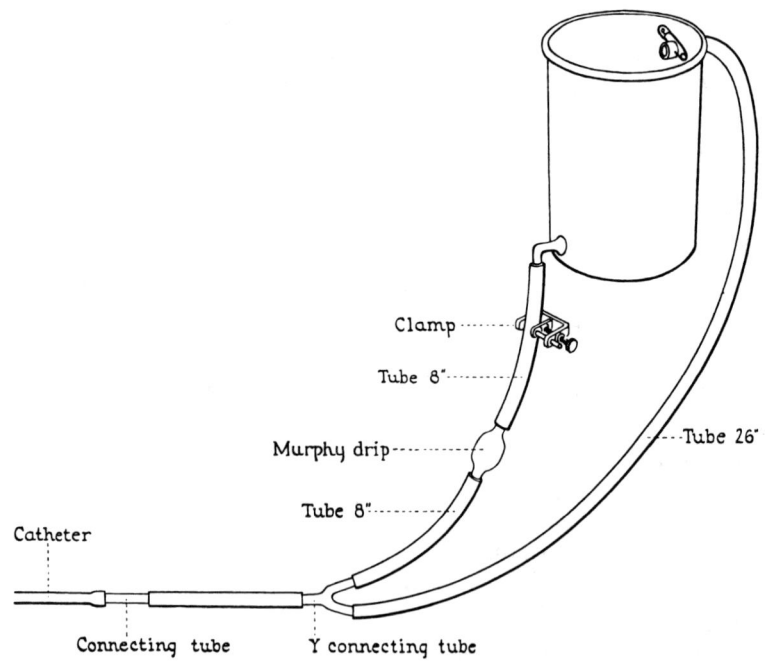

Solutions usually ordered
1. Tap water.
2. Physiological salt solution.
3. Glucose solution 5 per cent, and sodium bicarbonate solution, 2–5 per cent.

Preparation of equipment
1. Prepare can and tubing according to diagram.
2. Prepare solution ordered at 105° F.
3. Place articles on tray and carry with standard to bedside.

Preparation of patient
1. Tell patient what the treatment is to be.
2. Screen completely, if in a ward; if in a room, place screen before door.
3. Place patient in a comfortable position.
4. Replace covers with bath blanket.
5. Place bedpan cover and rubber protector under patient.

Procedure
1. Hang the can on the standard about 2 feet above the bed.
2. Attach the catheter and lubricate about 6 inches of it.
3. Open stopcock and fill tube with the warm solution.
4. Close stopcock and, following directions in previous demonstration, introduce the tube 4–6 inches.
5. If patient is restless, secure the tube by winding a narrow strip of adhesive 10 inches long once around catheter and fasten ends to either hip.
6. Establish drip, 40–60 drops a minute. Watch the tube for a few minutes to see whether the solution is being absorbed. Regulate accordingly.
7. Remove bath blanket and pull up upper bedclothes.
8. The treatment may be continuous or it may be stopped every 2 or 3 hours.
9. When discontinuing for a short time, the flow may be stopped by the stopcock. If for 2 hours or longer withdraw tube, disconnect, and clean.

After-care of patient
1. While treatment is being continued, note frequently whether solution is being absorbed.
2. Keep patient dry.
3. When treatment is finally discontinued, remove catheter, disconnect, and place in kidney basin.
4. Remove rubber protector and cover.
5. Leave patient dry and comfortable and unit in order.
6. Remove screen.
7. Remove articles to service room.

After-care of equipment
1. Rinse irrigating can and tubing with warm water. Leave stopcock open.
2. Force cold water through catheter. Be sure that all fecal matter is removed. If necessary, use applicator. Wash with soap and warm water in kidney basin.
3. Wash kidney basin.
4. Place irrigating can and tubing, kidney basin, and catheter in sterilizer. Boil 3 minutes.
5. Remove from sterilizer, dry glassware, and rinse rubber material in cold water and dry.
6. Set up can and tubing, wrap in towel, and replace on shelf.
7. Wash, dry, and replace basin.
8. Wash and dry rubber protector and replace in space provided.
9. Wash and dry hands.

Record
1. In treatment and medication column: time treatment started, kind, strength of solution, amount, time discontinued.
2. Record amounts on slip on chart (see below).
3. In nurse's remarks column: discomfort caused by treatment.
4. On temperature sheet: total amount taken during 24 hours, recorded in proper space by night nurse.
5. All charting is followed by nurse's initials.

SAMPLE OF SLIP ON CHART

Name.. Date..					
Time on	Time off	Amount Put in Can	Amount Left in Can	Amount Expelled	Amount Taken

References
Harmer, *Principles and Practice of Nursing*, pp. 646–49.
Kelley, *Textbook of Nursing Technique*, pp. 126–30.

VII. LOCAL APPLICATIONS OF HEAT AND COLD

Fomentations

Purpose
1. To relieve pain and congestion in the adjoining parts.
2. To relieve pain and congestion in the internal organs.
3. To relieve tympanites.
4. To reduce a swelling.
5. To stimulate the absorption of exudates.

General instructions
1. Avoid chilling the part before, during, or after the treatment.
2. Apply one fomentation as the other is removed.
3. Do not use turpentine in fomentations applied for the relief of pain or congestion of the kidneys.
4. Use great care to prevent the skin being burned.
5. Be sure medication is entirely removed and that area is dry after treatment is discontinued.
6. Be sure that flannel is wrung dry to prevent burning.
7. Rubber protector does not touch the skin.

Types
1. Abdominal.
2. Local.
3. Breast.

APPLIED TO ABDOMEN

Necessary articles
Tray.
Hand basin.
Stupe wringer and sticks.
2 pieces of flannel twice the size of the area.
Safety pins.
Piece of oiled muslin or waxed paper.
Olive oil, 2 drams in medicine glass.
Cotton applicators.
Castile or Ivory soap.
Small basin.
Kidney basin.
Cotton balls.
Hot-water bottle and cover.
Binder, triangular bandage, bandage, or bath towel, depending on area to be treated.

Preparation of equipment
1. Put stick through each side of stupe wringer.

2. Place one flannel in stupe wringer.
3. Place stupe wringer in sterilizer with sticks hanging outside, and heat until material has become thoroughly hot and steaming.
4. Remove wringer from sterilizer and wring flannels dry by twisting wringer with the sticks.
5. Remove sticks.
6. Warm basin and place stupe wringer with flannel in basin.
7. Fold wringer over so that heat will be retained in flannels.
8. Cover basin with oiled muslin or waxed paper, dry flannel and towel, and place on tray.
9. Place medicine glass with olive oil and cotton applicators in kidney basin.
10. Cover tray and carry with bath blanket to bedside.

Preparation of patient
1. Tell patient what the treatment is to be.
2. Screen completely.
3. Fanfold top bedding down to pubis and replace with bath blanket folded crosswise over chest.
4. Slip towel over abdomen and under gown.
5. Fold gown back over chest.
6. Place oiled muslin or waxed paper across chest.
7. Pass binder under patient.

Procedure
1. Fold back towel and apply warm olive oil to the area with the cotton applicators.*
2. Remove wet flannel from wringer, shake to incorporate air, and apply to area.
3. Cover with oiled muslin or waxed paper and then with dry flannel.
4. Fasten binder.
5. Fold down gown.
6. Pull top bedding up.
7. The second fomentation is prepared in the same way, before the first one is removed.
8. Renew in 15 minutes or as often as ordered.
9. Renew olive oil before every third application.

After-care of patient: when fomentations are discontinued
1. Bring to bedside on tray the additional equipment: cotton balls, soap, and small basin of warm water.

* If a turpentine fomentation, prepare solution as follows: Mix turpentine and oil in a medicine glass (1 dram of turpentine to 7 drams of olive oil), heat by letting stand in a basin of hot water. Stir mixture well before applying. Apply in the same way as the olive oil. This mixture is renewed before every third application according to the reddening of the skin.

2. Fanfold top bedding down to pubis.
3. Fold gown back over chest.
4. Loosen binder.
5. Fold dry flannel back over chest.
6. Remove wet flannel and rubber and place in basin.
7. Sponge area with cotton, soap, and water.
8. Pat thoroughly dry with towel and apply dry flannel.
9. Fasten binder.
10. Fold down gown.
11. Pull top bedding up and remove bath blanket.
12. Leave patient comfortable and unit in order.
13. Remove screen.
14. Carry tray to service room.

After-care of equipment
1. Stupe wringer and flannels are put with soiled linen.
2. Throw cotton balls and applicators with refuse.
3. Wash and dry oiled muslin and put away in space provided; waxed paper can be thrown away.
4. Boil basins, wash, dry, and replace on shelf.
5. Wash tray and replace on shelf.

APPLIED FOR PURELY LOCAL EFFECT

Types
1. Infected finger.
2. Boil, etc.

Application
1. Principle is the same as above.
2. Application should not be larger than necessary.
3. Olive oil omitted.
4. Held in place with bath towel, bandage, or triangular bandage.

APPLIED TO BREAST

Application
1. Principle the same as above.
2. Cut a hole in center of stupe cloths to prevent nipple being covered.
3. Held in place with a breast binder.

Record
1. In treatment and medication column: time, type, purpose, how long continued, reaction or results, initials.
2. In nurse's remarks column: general effect, comfort or discomfort.

References
Kelley, *Textbook of Nursing Technique*, pp. 163-64.

Harmer, *Principles and Practice of Nursing,* pp. 255–60.
Apple, "Hot Wet Packs and Stupes," *American Journal of Nursing,* 1933, p. 865.

Flaxseed Poultice

Purpose
1. To relieve pain and congestion in pneumonia.
2. To stimulate the absorption of inflammatory products in pneu
monia.
3. To hasten suppuration in infections.

General instructions
1. Have poultice as light as possible.
2. Have poultice as hot as can be borne by patient without burning.
3. Avoid exposure of part during or after treatment.
4. Never permit poultice to remain on longer than an hour.
5. Be sure that poultice is large enough to cover the area completely.

Necessary articles
Tray.
Boiling water⎫ amount depends on size of poultice.
Flaxseed   ⎭
Gauze, thin muslin, or any soft material double the size of fin-
ished poultice.
Piece of oiled muslin or waxed paper.
Board or heavy paper.
Saucepan and large spoon or spatula for preparation.
Flannel twice the size of area.
Sodium bicarbonate.
Binder, triangular bandage, bandage, or bath towel, depending
on the area to be treated.
Safety pins.
Olive oil, 2 drams in medicine glass.
Small basin.
Kidney basin.
Cotton applicators.
Castile or Ivory soap.
Cotton balls.

Preparation of equipment
1. Put water on to boil.
2. Spread a towel on the board or heavy paper.
3. Place flannel, oiled muslin, and thin muslin (fold as for mustard plaster).

4. When water is boiling, add flaxseed to it, stirring mixture with a spoon or spatula.
5. Make mixture just thick enough to drop from spoon.
6. When it is the right consistency, remove from fire and add 1 teaspoonful of sodium bicarbonate. Beat until light.
7. Spread it evenly on the muslin foundation about ½ inch thick.
8. Fold sides of muslin to meet center and fold one end into the other.
9. Roll together the flannel, oiled muslin, and poultice.
10. Wash articles used in preparation.
11. Carry with other articles on a tray to bedside.

Preparation of patient
1. Tell patient what the treatment is to be.
2. Screen completely, if in a ward; if in a room, place screen before door.
3. Arrange bedding and gown so they will be out of the way.
4. Place binder underneath the part to be poulticed.

Procedure
1. Apply warm olive oil to part with cotton applicators. Place soiled applicators at opposite end of basin from clean ones.
2. Apply poultice slowly so as to accustom patient to the heat.
3. Cover with oiled muslin and flannel.
4. Fasten binder to hold poultice in place.
5. Change every hour or as ordered.

Procedure of changing
1. Make fresh poultice exactly as first.
2. Roll in towel and carry to bedside.
3. Unfasten binder and slip used poultice from underneath oiled muslin.

After-care of patient
1. Bring to bedside on tray the additional equipment: cotton balls, soap, and small basin of warm water.
2. Arrange bedding and gown so they will be out of the way.
3. Unfasten binder.
4. Fold flannel back.
5. Remove poultice and oiled muslin and place on tray.
6. Sponge area with cotton, soap, and water.
7. Pat thoroughly dry with towel and apply dry flannel.
8. Fasten binder.
9. Leave patient comfortable and unit in order.
10. Remove screen.
11. Carry tray to service room.

After-care of equipment
1. Throw cotton balls, applicators, and poultice with refuse.
2. Wash and dry oiled muslin and put away in space provided; waxed paper can be thrown away.
3. Boil kidney basin, wash, dry, and replace on shelf.
4. Wash medicine glass, dry, and put away.
5. Wash tray and replace on shelf.

Record
1. In treatment and medication column: time, type of treatment, area to which applied, how long continued.
2. In nurse's remarks column: reactions to treatment.
3. Nurse's initials follow charting in each column.

References
Harmer, *Principles and Practice of Nursing*, pp. 260–63.
Kelley, *Textbook of Nursing Technique*, pp. 163–65.

Mustard Plaster or Sinapism

Purpose
1. To relieve cerebral congestion, headache, and neuralgia, or congestion in pleurisy and pneumonia.
2. To relieve nausea and pain in the stomach.
3. To relieve pain in the abdomen caused by flatulence and congestion.

Necessary articles
Tray.
Mustard.
Flour.
Dish and spoon.
Tepid water.
Gauze, thin muslin, or any other soft material double the size of finished plaster.
Face towel.
Hot-water bottle, warm plate, or warm basin.
Cotton balls.
Castile or Ivory soap.
Olive oil, 2 drams in medicine glass.
Cotton applicators.

Preparation of equipment
1. Fold face towel in quarters.
2. To fold muslin: fold over one end; fold sides to center; original ends to center, putting unfolded end into folded end; crease edges (this shows the size of plaster). Open up and place on towel.

3. Prepare plaster by mixing mustard and flour as follows:
   For adult: 1 part mustard to 6 parts flour.
   For child: 1 part mustard to 12 parts flour.
4. Mix slowly with tepid water.
5. Mix well to insure that there are no lumps of mustard.
6. Make a paste thick enough to spread without running.
7. Spread paste about ¼ inch thick on muslin inside of creased area.
8. Refold muslin as stated above.
9. Place the plaster, smooth side down, on a hot-water bottle, warm plate, or warm basin and cover with face towel.
10. Carry plaster with other articles to bedside on a small tray.

Preparation of patient
1. Tell patient what the treatment is to be.
2. Screen completely, if in a ward; if in a room, place screen before door.
3. Arrange bedclothing and gown so that they will be out of the way.

Procedure
1. With cotton applicators apply warm olive oil to the part. Place soiled applicators at opposite end of basin from clean ones.
2. Apply plaster to skin and cover with face towel.
3. Leave 15 or 20 minutes or until the skin is well reddened.
4. Watch the skin closely after 5 minutes have elapsed; a burn from a mustard application is invariably the result of carelessness.

After-care of patient
1. Bring to bedside on tray the additional equipment: cotton balls, soap, and small basin of warm water.
2. Remove plaster and towel and place on tray.
3. Sponge area with cotton, soap, and water.
4. Pat thoroughly dry with towel.
5. Replace bedding and gown.
6. Leave patient comfortable and unit in order.
7. Remove screen.

After-care of equipment
1. Throw cotton balls, applicators, and plaster with refuse.
2. Put towel with soiled linen.
3. Boil basin, wash, dry, and replace on shelf.
4. Wash medicine glass, dry, and put away.
5. Wash tray and replace on shelf.

Record
1. In treatment and medication column: time, nature of treatment, area to which applied, duration.
2. In nurse's remarks column: reaction to or effects of, such as relief of tympanites, pain, or nausea.
3. Nurse's initials follow charting in each column.

References
Harmer, *Principles and Practice of Nursing,* pp. 263–64.
Kelley, *Textbook of Nursing Technique,* pp. 165–67.
Pope, *Practical Nursing,* pp. 492–95.

The Hot Foot Bath *

Purpose
1. To relieve congestion in remote or local parts.
2. To relieve, prevent, or break up a cold.
3. To relieve pelvic congestion.

Necessary articles
Foot tub half full of water 110–120° F., or temperature ordered.
Bath blanket.
2 bath towels.
Hot-water bottle and cover.
Rubber sheet.
Pitcher of hot water.
Bath thermometer.

Preparation of equipment
1. Assemble bath blanket, rubber sheet, and bath towels.
2. Prepare tub or water at correct temperature. Test with bath thermometer.
3. Carry articles to bedside.

Preparation of patient
1. Tell patient what the treatment is going to be.
2. Screen completely, if in a ward; if in a room, place screen before door.
3. Loosen upper bedclothes at foot of bed.
4. Flex patient's knees.
5. Fold back upper covers approximately 2 feet from lower edge of the mattress, being sure that the patient's feet are kept covered.
6. Place rubber drawsheet across foot of bed.
7. Place folded bath blanket on rubber sheet, folded edge even with foot of mattress. Fanfold top half back.
8. Place bath towel across bath blanket.

* Moving pictures have been made of this procedure. See Preface, page iv.

9. Raise patient's feet and legs with arm nearest head of bed and draw rubber sheet, bath blanket, and towel under feet.
10. Fold back upper bedclothes to knees, pulling up bath blanket at same time.

Procedure

1. Place tub lengthwise near the feet.
2. Fold back corner of blanket.
3. Put your arm nearest head of bed under patient's legs and your hand under his heels.
4. Put other arm across tub, grasp it on far side, and move it forward into position at the same time that you raise the feet and legs from the bed. This is done under the top layer of the blanket, the arm being kept across the tub to prevent the blanket getting into the water.
5. Place patient's feet in the tub slowly, heels first.
6. Place second bath towel, folded, over rim of tub between patient's legs and tub.
7. Bring rubber sheet up over blanket and knees.
8. Fold top covers down over foot of bed. Do not tuck in.
9. The feet are kept in the water from 15 to 20 minutes.
10. If it is necessary to raise the temperature of the water, pour in hot water from the pitcher slowly, keeping your hand between the patient's legs and the stream. This can be done without uncovering the tub anywhere except at the point where you are pouring in the water.
11. When ready to remove tub, prepare hot-water bottle and bring to bedside.
12. To remove tub, turn covers back above the knees.
13. Put your arm under the legs as when putting the feet in tub.
14. Pull tub toward you and place the feet on the bath towel.
15. Remove tub.
16. Dry the feet with bath towel under the feet.
17. Remove blanket and rubber sheet and pull down upper covers.

After-care of patient

1. Place hot-water bottle at the feet.
2. Tuck covers under mattress.
3. Leave patient comfortable and unit in order.
4. Remove articles to service room.

After-care of equipment

1. Wash and boil tub, dry, and replace on shelf.
2. Wash rubber sheet and hot-water bottle, dry, and replace in space provided.
3. Dry pitcher and replace on shelf.

Record
1. In treatment and medication column: time, treatment, duration.
2. In nurse's remarks column: results, if observable.

References
Reid, Hoffman, Jennings, and Read, *A Manual of Nursing Procedures*, pp. 89–91.
Kelley, *Textbook of Nursing Technique*, pp. 73–74.
Sanders, *Modern Methods in Nursing*, p. 98.
Harmer, *Principles and Practice of Nursing*, pp. 264–65.

Cold Compresses for the Head

Purpose
1. To relieve congestion or pain in the head.
2. To reduce temperature.

General instructions
1. Avoid allowing the water to drop from the compresses.
2. Do not allow patient to become chilled.

Necessary articles
A medium-sized basin used the same as for eye compresses.
Piece of ice about size of basin, flat on top.
Face towel.
Rubber protector.
2 compresses 8x4 inches made of 4 thicknesses of loosely woven cotton material. Fold with raw edges turned in.
Tray.

Preparation of equipment
1. Cover basin with piece of gauze.
2. Make gauze taut by tying a string or another piece of gauze around top edge of basin.
3. Place ice on gauze.
4. Wet the 2 compresses, wring out as dry as possible, and place on ice.
5. Place basin, face towel, and rubber protector on tray.
6. Carry tray to bedside.

Preparation of patient
1. Screen completely.
2. Cover rubber protector with towel and place under the patient's head.
3. Be sure patient's hair is brushed well away from forehead.

Procedure
1. Place a compress from the ice across the forehead close to the eyes, but not over them.

2. Change compresses every 5 minutes.

3. Continue for 30 minutes or as directed.

After-care of patient

1. Remove last compress and drop into basin.

2. Remove towel and rubber protector and place on tray.

3. Remove screen and leave patient comfortable and unit in order.

4. Carry tray to service room.

After-care of equipment

1. Wash and dry basin and replace on shelf.

2. Put rubber protector and tray in place provided.

3. Put towel with soiled linen.

Record

1. In treatment and medication column: time, type of treatment, area, purpose, how long applied, effects, nurse's initials.

2. In nurse's remarks column: general effect, restlessness relieved, sleep induced.

References

Harmer, *Principles and Practice of Nursing*, p. 282.

ADVANCED PROCEDURES

I. THE ADMINISTRATION OF MEDICINES

Purpose

1. To impress upon the student the importance of intelligent, conscientious, and accurate administration of medications.
2. To impress upon the student that the administration of medicines is one of the greatest responsibilities assigned to her.
3. To teach her that it is essential to have a working knowledge of pharmacology and metrology.

General instructions

1. The administration of medicines is one of the greatest responsibilities assigned to student nurses.
2. No nurse should be ignorant, uninterested, or mechanical in the administration of drugs.
3. Nurses only are responsible for the passing and administering of all medications.
4. Nurses should see that medications are received by the patient promptly, accurately, and in such a way as to give best results.
5. To administer drugs intelligently, the nurse should know and consider.
   a. The nature of the drug.
   b. To what its action, both local and systemic, is due.
   c. The maximum and minimum dosage.
   d. The factors that modify dosage and its effect:
      (1) Age.
      (2) Sex.
      (3) Previous habits or toleration.
      (4) Idiosyncrasy.
      (5) Temperament and occupation.
      (6) Condition of patient.
      (7) Nature and form of medication.
      (8) Object of medication.
      (9) Time of administration.
      (10) Channel of administration.
   e. The disease from which patient is suffering.
   f. The effect desired.
   g. Why the drug is being given.
   h. The symptoms that indicate the desired and possible undesired results.
   i. Symptoms of overdosing.
   j. The effect of habit-forming drugs and the necessity for and means of restricting their use.

Channels of administration
1. By mouth.
2. By rectum: suppositories.
3. By inhalation: tr. benzoin, steam.
4. Externally: lotions and ointments.
5. By hypodermic injection.
   a. Subcutaneously: Pantapon.
   b. Intracutaneously: Schick test.
   c. Intramuscularly: Bismogenol.
   d. Intravenously: Glucose.
   e. Intraspinally: Meningococcic serum.

Care of medications and medicine cabinet
1. *Medicine cabinet must be kept locked.* Never leave the key in the lock.
2. Arrange drugs in medicine cupboard with bottles of the same size together; keep all the more powerful drugs separate from others and in bottles having a rough exterior or other distinguishing feature and marked "poison."
3. Keep oils in a cool place.
4. Keep vaccines in icebox.
5. Never change the label on a bottle; have the druggist do it.
6. Keep labels clean.
7. Keep shelves and bottles clean.
8. Keep all bottles corked tightly. Those that contain volatile substances will become either stronger or weaker if left uncorked.
9. Any change in color, odor, or consistency of medicines should be reported and a fresh supply obtained.
10. Report shortage of drugs to head nurse.
11. Return special prescriptions to Drug Room when medicine is discontinued.
12. Never order a large amount of drugs; some deteriorate.
13. No medicine is to be kept in the medicine cupboard in a medicine glass.

Rules for administration of medicines
1. When preparing and giving medications, concentrate on what is being done and allow no conversation or interruption.
2. Always give *exactly* what is ordered and *on time*.
3. Give *minims* when *minims* are ordered, *drops* when *drops* are ordered.
4. Read the label on the bottle *three times*.
   a. Before taking from the shelf.
   b. Before pouring from the bottle.
   c. After pouring from the bottle.
5. Always shake bottle before pouring out liquid medicine.

6. While pouring medicine hold bottle with label on upper side to avoid defacing it. Before replacing bottle, wipe rim with gauze kept for that purpose.
7. While pouring, hold glass on level with eye, with thumbnail on mark of quantity required.
8. Never allow one patient to carry medicines to another.
9. Never use medicine about the contents of which you are in doubt, nor medicine from an unmarked bottle.
10. When patients refuse to take medicine, it must be reported and recorded on chart.
11. Remember that there is an element of danger in every drop of medicine.
12. Never prepare or give a drug in the dark or in a dim light.
13. Never give a medicine about which you have a shadow of doubt as to the dosage or effect; find out about it.
14. Medicines are to be given as soon as prepared.
15. The nurse who prepares the medicine always gives it and remains with the patient to see that it is taken; if refused, report it to the head nurse and record.
16. All p. r. n. orders must be approved by the head nurse or night supervisor.

THE MEDICINE CARD SYSTEM

Purpose
1. To provide a system of marking medications while pouring.

General instructions
1. Cards must be clean and legible.
2. Cards must be accurate.
3. Medication to be given by hypodermic injections must be designated on the ticket.
4. Full name is to be used on the card.
5. To make out a card:
    (1) Cards are made out by the nurse instructed to do so from the doctor's order book in accordance with the routine of the hospital.
    (2) Card is then left on head nurse's desk.
    (3) Head nurse or night supervisor checks card with order book, marks card O. K. with her initials, and places it in medicine card box.
    (4) Sample of card:

```
+------------------------------+
|       Mr. John Brown         |
|  Tr. Digitalis — MV —t. i. d.|
|          8 — 12 — 5          |
|  5-1-34          O. K. H. T. |
+------------------------------+
```

6. To discontinue a card:
    (1) When medication is discontinued, card is bent by nurse instructed to do so and left on head nurse's desk.
    (2) Head nurse or night supervisor checks card with order book and destroys card.
7. Key to colors of cards:
    (1) Q. 3 h. — Pink — 9, 12, 3, 6, etc.
    (2) Q. 4 h. & Q. i. d. — Red — 8, 12, 4, etc., and 8, 12, 4, 8.
    (3) A. C. t. i. d. — Blue — ½ hour before meals.
    (4) P. C. t. i. d. — Yellow — ½ hour after meals.
    (5) Irregular — Green.
    (6) Treatment — White.
    (7) Q. h. — Green, one corner off.
    (8) Q. 2 h. — Red, one corner off — 6, 8, 10, etc.
    (9) Q. 6 h. — Blue, one corner off — 6, 12, etc.
    (10) B. i. d. — Yellow, one corner off — 8 A. M., 4 P. M. or 8 P. M.

ADMINISTRATION OF MEDICINES BY MOUTH

Purpose
1. To give medications by mouth so as to insure as completely correct and full effect as possible.
2. To give irritating or unpalatable medication in such a way as to lessen the discomfort.
3. To give medications in such a way as to insure correct dosage.

General instructions
1. Make the dose as palatable as possible.
2. Never record a dose as given until patient has taken it.
3. If water is necessary with the medicine, the nurse should see that it is provided. Use either very hot or very cold water.
4. Stand by any patient who must be awakened and see that the medicine is taken.
5. Do not leave bedside until medicine is taken.
6. When giving liquid medicine to an unconscious patient, drop it far back on the tongue, using a dessert spoon.
7. Never place a pill or powder on the tongue of a delirious or unconscious patient; dissolve it in water before giving.
8. Tablets are never poured into the hand: pour required number into lid of bottle or, if bottle has a cork, hold cork against rim of bottle until required number of tablets are in neck of bottle, then permit them to drop into medicine glass.

Preparation of equipment
1. Wash hands.

2. Refer to Kardex or medication sheet to find out what medications are to be given.
3. Secure medicine cards; be sure you have all of them.
4. Place card on shelf; read name and medication.
5. Find medicine on shelf; take bottle from shelf in right hand, shake it, and read label the first time. Compare label with card.
6. Remove cork with thumb and first and second fingers.
7. Hold cork between first and second fingers.
8. Hold medicine glass in left hand so that the mark of the prescribed amount is on a level with the eye.
9. Pour in enough drug to reach the line designating the prescribed amount. Read label second time.
10. Wipe rim of bottle, replace cork, and replace bottle on shelf. Read label third time.
11. Dilute medication to approximately ½ ounce unless contraindicated.
12. Read label on medication card and place card with medicine glass and medicine glass on tray.
13. Pour all medications in same way.
14. Carry medication tray to ward.

Procedure
1. Note name on patient's bed.
2. Speak patient's name and secure affirmative response from him.
3. Read name and medication on card.
4. Give medication which has previously been diluted. If patient wishes, give more water. Remove card and place face down on tray.
5. Continue until all medications have been given.

After-care of equipment
1. Replace cards in proper places.
2. Take medicine glasses to kitchen, wash with warm water and soap, dry well, wipe off medicine tray, wash pitcher, replace glasses and pitcher, and take tray back to medicine cabinet. Leave medicine cabinet immaculate.

Record
1. In treatment and medication column: time, name of preparation, dosage, channel of administration if other than oral; if given by a doctor, state his name.
2. In nurse's remarks column: purpose (if known by nurse) and effects if observable.
3. Initials follow all recording.

References

Blumgarten, *Textbook of Materia Medica*, pp. 115–35.
Goostray, *Introduction to Materia Medica*, pp. 145–52.
Harmer, *Principles and Practice of Nursing*, pp. 490–501.
Muse, *Materia Medica, Pharmacology and Therapeutics*, pp. 18–34.

Administration of Suppositories

Purpose
1. To introduce drugs into the rectum for a direct local effect.

Kinds of suppositories
1. Concentrated food.
2. Soap.
3. Glycerine.
4. Plain or medicated cocoa butter.

Necessary articles
Suppository.
Gauze squares.
Tube of vaseline.
Finger cot or rectal tube.

Preparation of equipment
1. Secure suppository.
2. Place a very small amount of lubricant on gauze square and place suppository on square.
3. Carry with other articles on a tray to bedside.

Preparation of patient
1. Tell patient what the treatment is to be.
2. Screen completely, if in a ward; if in a room, place screen before door.
3. Turn patient on left side if possible; otherwise she may be in the dorsal recumbent position.
4. If patient is on her side, fold covers back, exposing only the area necessary.
5. If patient is on her back, drape as for external douche.

Procedure
1. Cover index finger with finger cot. Lubricate finger.
2. Pass suppository into the rectum beyond the internal sphincter muscle. The suppository can be pushed in with a rectal tube instead of using finger with finger cot.
3. Apply pressure over the anus for a few moments until the patient has no desire to expel the suppository.

After-care of patient
1. Leave patient comfortable and unit in order.

After-care of equipment
1. Wash and boil finger cot or rectal tube, dry, and put away.

Record
1. In medication and treatment column: time, name of preparation, dosage, purpose (if known by nurse).
2. In nurse's remarks column: general systemic or local effect, if observable.
3. Initials follow all recording.

References:
Harmer, *Principles and Practice of Nursing*, pp. 501–03.
Kelley, *Textbook of Nursing Technique*, pp. 91–92.

Inunctions

Purpose
1. To administer a drug through the skin.

Medications most commonly applied
1. Cod-liver oil.
2. Olive oil.
3. Cocoa butter.
4. Mercurial ointment.

Necessary articles for applying cod-liver oil, olive oil, or cocoa butter
Wash basin containing warm water.
Soap.
Bath towel.
Medication.

Areas to which application may be made
Chest, abdomen, back, limbs, whole body.

Preparation of equipment
1. Prepare articles, warm the oil, place on tray, and carry to bedside.

Preparation of patient
1. Tell patient what the treatment is to be.
2. Screen completely, if in a ward; if in a room, place screen before door.
3. Expose area and place bath towel in position.

Procedure
1. Cleanse skin with warm water and soap and dry.
2. Rub oil in with palm of hand until absorbed.
3. Use a circular motion.

After-care of patient
1. Replace bedding; leave patient comfortable and unit in order.

After-care of equipment
1. Wash and boil basin and container used for oil.
2. Replace articles in space provided.

Record
1. In treatment and medication space: time, name of preparation, dosage, channel of administration, place given.
2. Nurse's initials follow all recording.

References
Kelley, *Textbook of Nursing Technique*, p. 91.
Harmer, *Principles and Practice of Nursing*, pp. 507–08.

APPLICATION OF MERCURIAL OINTMENT

Necessary articles
Wash basin containing warm water.
Soap.
Bath towel.
Medication.
Rubber glove.
Piece of old muslin to wipe ointment from glove.
Newspaper.

Preparation of equipment
1. Prepare articles and place on tray.
2. Consult head nurse or chart in regard to portions of body that are used for the "course" of treatments.
3. Carry tray to bedside.

Preparation of patient
1. Tell patient what the treatment is to be.
2. Screen completely, if in a ward; if in a room, place screen before door.
3. Expose portion of body to be treated.
4. Protect bed with newspaper.

Procedure
1. Put on rubber glove and apply ointment to exposed area.
2. Rub it into skin thoroughly by using a rotary motion.
3. Apply ointment in this way for 5 days, using a different surface each day.
4. Do not give treatment on sixth day.
5. Give patient a bath on seventh day and then continue the treatment as before.

After-care of patient
1. Remove paper and cover area.
2. Leave patient comfortable and unit in order.

3. Remove screen.
4. Carry out tray.

After-care of equipment
1. Wash rubber glove in soap and water, dry, and powder.
2. Wash and boil basin.
3. Replace articles in space provided.

Record
1. In treatment and medication column: time, name of preparation, dosage, channel of administration, place given.
2. Nurse's initials follow all recording.

References
Harmer, *Principles and Practice of Nursing*, pp. 507–08.
Kelley, *Textbook of Nursing Technique*, p. 91.

Inhalations

Purpose
1. To relieve spasmodic breathing.
2. To disinfect bronchial secretions.
3. To stimulate expectoration.
4. To give comfort to the patient.

General instructions
1. If patient is up and about, all steam inhalations should be given at bedtime. If treatment is ordered during the day, patient should not be permitted to go out for at least an hour afterward.
2. Avoid drafts.
3. Whatever method is used, great care must be taken that patient is not burned.
4. If a canopy is used, arrange it so that there will be ample ventilation and so that it will present a neat appearance.
5. Steam inhalations are usually given for 10 or 15 minutes every 4 hours or continuously.

Medications most commonly used
1. Aromatic spirits of ammonia:
   a. Saturate a piece of gauze and hold to patient's nose.
   b. Usually given in syncope.
2. Amyl nitrite pearls:
   a. Never given without a doctor's order.
   b. Given as a stimulant.
   c. Crush pearl in a piece of gauze and allow patient to inhale vapor.
   d. Care must be taken not to hold too close to the nose, as it may cause epistaxis.

3. Stramonium leaves:
   a. Given as dry inhalation.
   b. The drug is placed on a heated plate and fumes are inhaled through a cone.

STEAM, METHOD NO. 1

Necessary articles
Inhalator.
Cone or canopy.

Preparation of equipment
1. Prepare inhalator by filling container with water.
2. Attach plug to electric fixture near bedside and turn on.
3. Attach frame, if available, to head of bed.
4. Cover.

Procedure
1. When steam appears, place goose neck through canopy in such a position that steam will fill the tent, but will not be near patient. If there is no canopy, the cone is used.
2. Be sure that there is absolutely no danger to patient from inhalation before leaving room.
3. Watch patient closely.

After-care of patient
1. Remove canopy and inhalator.
2. Be sure that patient is not in a draft.
3. Leave warm, dry, and comfortable.
4. Should remain in bed for at least an hour after treatment.

After-care of equipment
1. Clean inhalator and return to place provided.
2. Put sheet with soiled laundry.
3. Put frame in place provided.

Record
1. In treatment and medication column: time, treatment, duration.
2. In nurse's remarks column: effect, if observable, relief obtained, diaphoresis, etc.

References
Harmer, *Principles and Practice of Nursing*, pp. 508–11.
Kelley, *Textbook of Nursing Technique*, pp. 197–201.
Harser, "Moist Inhalation," *American Journal of Nursing*, 1931, p. 168.
Carey, "Improvised Equipment for Steam Inhalations," *American Journal of Nursing*, 1934, p. 249.

METHOD No. 2

Necessary articles

Bath blanket.
Medication.
Boiling water in pitcher.
Bath towel.
Face towel.
Large hand basin.

Preparation of equipment

1. Pour prescribed drug into pitcher of boiling water. (Always use an old pitcher.)
2. Cover with folded face towel.
3. Fold bath towel in thirds crosswise and wrap around pitcher so as to prevent patient from being burned and to form funnel through which vapor can be inhaled.
4. Place pitcher in basin, carry with other articles to bedside, and place on bedside table.

Preparation of patient

1. Fasten bath blanket around patient's shoulders.
2. Assist patient to one side of bed.
3. Place patient on his side with his head near the edge of pillows.

Procedure

1. Make canopy of face towel and place basin with pitcher in position so that patient can inhale steam.
2. Continue for approximately 10 minutes.
3. Patient should not be left alone during this time.
4. Remove articles to service room.

After-care of patient

1. See that patient is dry and comfortable and not in a draft.
2. Leave unit in order.

After-care of equipment

1. Place towels with soiled linen.
2. Wash pitcher and basin, dry, and replace on shelf.

Record

1. In treatment and medication column: time, treatment, duration.
2. In nurse's remarks column: effect, if observable, relief obtained, diaphoresis, etc.

References

"Improvised Equipment," *American Journal of Nursing*, 1933, p. 347.

Oxygen Tent

Purpose

1. To enable the patient to breathe cool air richer in oxygen content than air of atmosphere where the oxygen minute volume of the lungs fails to meet the body requirement.

Principle

1. To air of atmosphere, which is kept circulating by an electric motor, is constantly added pure oxygen at a definite known rate. This is usually about 6 liters a minute, which brings the oxygen percentage of the air to about 50. The air is cooled and dried by ice and lime, over which it flows, and the carbon dioxide is lost either through the seams of the tent or if necessary by contact with lime.

General instructions

1. See that tent is kept as airtight as possible. In back and at sides it is tucked between mattress and spring, and in front covered securely with spread. The patient's head must *always* be covered by the tent, since any change in oxygen pressure within the lungs causes serious danger to the patient.

2. Observe temperature within the tent frequently and maintain at the level indicated by the pathology service. This is usually between 65° and 70° F. When the temperature is above 70° F., the patient is apt to develop a sensation of suffocation and become very restless. The temperature may be regulated by the speed of the motor.

3. Keep patient's chest and shoulders covered with 2 blankets.

4. Observe the meters to see that there is oxygen in the tank and that the rate of flow remains that ordered by the pathologist. (The pathologist is responsible for ordering the tanks of oxygen from the Drug Room.)

5. Keep the ice chest full of medium-sized chunks of ice.

6. See that drain pan is emptied when necessary.

7. In caring for patient, use the armholes in sides of tent. Keep the sleeves folded twice and clipped when not in use.

8. See that visitors do not lift nor reach under tent.

9. If lime is used, the pathologist is responsible for its change as often as necessary.

10. When discontinued, note in the notebook attached to the tent the name of patient, the hour, and the amount of oxygen left in the tank.

11. When discontinued, wash inside and outside of tent with warm water and mild soap before returning it to storage.

12. No flames or sparks should be brought near the tent and one should not make any X-ray examination with portable X-ray

apparatus while tent is in place. During the winter it is advisable for the operator to touch another person or an object before touching the apparatus to guard against the possibility of static sparks.

13. The patient should not attempt to hold conversation while in the tent, since the exertion necessary to speaking loudly is dangerous for the patient.

14. The pathologist starts the tent, changes oxygen tanks, and discontinues the tent.

15. The head nurse notifies the pathologist:
    a. When the oxygen tank is nearly empty.
    b. When the rate of oxygen flow changes.
    c. When any unusual difficulty is encountered.

Record
1. Time started and by whom.
2. Time discontinued and by whom.
3. Temperature of air in tent every 2 hours.

References
"Maintenance Rules for Oxygen Therapy Equipment," *Modern Hospital,* July, 1933.

Wright, *Applied Physiology,* pp. 16, 270, 293, 343–45, 358–60, 365–68, 495.

Pamphlets distributed by Linde Air Products Company, including Ganash, *Recent Trends in Oxygen Therapy* and *The Widening Field of Oxygen Therapy,* and Barach and Richards, *Effects of Treatment with Oxygen in Cardiac Failure* (reprint).

Administration of Drugs Subcutaneously

Purpose
1. To obtain prompt action of a drug.
2. To prevent loss of drug in digestive tract when small dose is given.
3. To prevent irritation of lining of digestive tract by irritating drugs.
4. To avoid destruction of animal extracts and other types of medications by digestive juices and enzymes.

Necessary articles
Receptacle for sterile cotton pledgets.
Small bottle of alcohol 70 per cent.
Wide-mouthed glass-stoppered bottle of alcohol 70 per cent with 4 thicknesses of gauze in bottom.
Alcohol lamp.
Tablespoon.

Small forceps.
Small rubber bulb.
Hypodermic syringe.
Wire needle 25 gage, ¾ inch long.
Tablets or medications to be given.

Preparation of equipment

1. Wash hands. Read order in order book; make note of it on piece of scrap paper.
2. Obtain drug, read label carefully.
3. Remove wire from needle. Test by drawing across ball of thumb to see that point is sharp and without hooks and by forcing alcohol through it to see that lumen is open.
4. Draw barrel full of alcohol; leave plunger out; leave both in wide-mouthed bottle of alcohol.
5. Light alcohol lamp.
6. Place needle in tablespoon with point toward small part of spoon; cover with water.
7. Boil needle for 1 minute. Flame forceps at same time. Place forceps so that point remains sterile.
8. Put spoon down.
9. Remove barrel and plunger from alcohol; rinse with water from spoon.
10. Draw up 20–25 minims of water into syringe.
11. Pick up needle with forceps and attach to syringe.
12. Remove cotton ball from receptacle; pour alcohol on it from small bottle.
13. Wrap cotton ball around needle; place on table, letting end of syringe rest on table.
14. Empty water from spoon and flame sufficiently to get it dry. Extinguish flame.
15. Read label on medication. With aid of stopper on vial, place tablet in spoon. Read label and replace in box.
16. Force water from syringe into spoon and draw back and forth until tablet is dissolved.
17. Draw solution into syringe, being sure to get it all, and be sure needle is very secure.
18. Enfold needle in alcohol sponge.
19. Read order book again.
20. Carry to patient.

Preparation of patient

1. Tell patient what you are going to do.
2. Select site in which it is to be given; fold gown or bed clothing out of way.

3. If patient is a pre-operative, he should be lying down and other preparations all made before hypodermic is given.
4. When giving hypodermic at frequent intervals, alternate between right and left arm and right and left thigh.

Procedure
1. Disinfect skin with alcohol cotton ball and expel air by holding syringe with needle pointing upward.
2. Hold cotton ball between second and third fingers of left hand and pull skin tight.
3. Insert needle quickly at a 45° angle (do not insert to hilt), withdraw slightly, then inject fluid by pressure on piston with thumb.
4. Make pressure with sponge over point of puncture.
5. Withdraw needle quickly, wipe upward with cotton ball over spot.

After-care of equipment
1. Clean syringe and needle, filling and emptying with water and then alcohol. Take alcohol from wide-mouthed bottle and put back into bottle.
2. Dry needle thoroughly by blowing air through with rubber bulb 3 or 4 times.
3. Replace wire in needle and put in box.
4. Leave syringe separated and in container.
5. Wash spoon, if necessary scour it, and leave clean and dry.
6. Tray should be left in order at all times, with bottles filled and a supply of cotton balls.

Record
1. On narcotic sheet and check number as soon as given.
2. Check in doctor's order book as given, with time if a "stat" order.
3. Chart in medication and treatment column: time, medication, dose, location.
4. In nurse's remarks column: purpose and effect of medication.
5. All charting is followed by nurse's initials.

References
Harmer, *Principles and Practice of Nursing*, pp. 503–05.

Administration of Insulin

General instructions
1. Insulin is a solution of the anti-diabetic principle obtained from the islands of Langerhan in the pancreas.
2. Insulin should be kept in a cool place.
3. The strength is measured in units — 1.0 unit of insulin will usually enable the body to utilize from 1 to 2 grams of glucose.

Necessary articles

Insulin. Examine label closely to determine the strength of insulin contained. It is sold in 5 strengths, but those most commonly used are:

U 20, containing 20 units in 1 cc.

U 40, containing 40 units in 1 cc. This strength is preferable if a single dosage is more than 20 units.

Syringe. The insulin syringe is graduated in insulin units to a total quantity of 1 cc. There are two scales, one to be used when unit 20 insulin is measured and another for unit 40 insulin. Care must be taken to use the scale that corresponds to the strength of insulin used. Other equipment is the same as for any hypodermic injection.

Preparation of equipment and dosage

1. The needle, syringe, and forceps are prepared as for other hypodermic injections.
2. As soon as forceps have been prepared, a cotton ball wet with 70 per cent alcohol is placed on rubber cap of insulin vial.
3. Special precaution must be taken to rinse *all* the alcohol from the barrel and plunger, for alcohol renders insulin impotent.
4. Join needle to syringe.
5. Wipe off cap of vial with the alcohol cotton ball that has been placed upon it. Discard the cotton ball. Draw into syringe an amount of air equal to the amount of insulin to be given.
6. Grasping the hub of the needle between the thumb and forefinger, pierce the depression in the center of the cap, pushing the needle forward in a straight line.
7. Inject the air into the air space in the vial. This prevents the formation of a vacuum in the vial, which would cause difficulty in withdrawing an accurate amount of insulin. If air is injected into the insulin, bubbles are apt to be formed.
8. Invert the vial and withdraw the required dose, plus a minute additional amount to cover loss in expelling air before administration.

Procedure

1. Prepare site of injection as for other hypodermic injections. Shift the site used, using both arms and both thighs.
2. Inject the insulin deeply into the subcutaneous tissue, but not intramuscularly. (Needle should be in freely movable tissue.) Injection should be made very slowly. After removal of the needle, massage the surrounding tissue thoroughly (teach patient to do this) to stimulate absorption of the insulin and to prevent the development of areas of induration and fibrosis caused by acute or chronic irritating effect of the drug.

After-care of patient

1. Insulin reaction may occur shortly after administration or may be delayed for several hours. (The maximum effect of insulin is reached from a half hour to several hours after the administration, depending upon the dose.) Symptoms include feeling of hunger, sudden weakness, perspiration, staring expression, and possibly mental disturbances and convulsions, stupor and unconsciousness. If these symptoms appear, the doctor is notified immediately in order that glucose in some form may be promptly administered.

Record

1. Chart as for any hypodermic injection.

References

Wright, *Applied Physiology.*

Diabetes Mellitus, manual published by Eli Lilly and Co.

Insulin, information sheet accompanying insulin.

II. EYE, EAR, NOSE, AND THROAT TREATMENTS

Administration of Eye Drops

Purpose
1. To dilate the pupil.
2. To contract the pupil.
3. To relieve inflammatory conditions of the eye.
4. To produce local anesthesia preparatory to operation.
5. To treat certain eye infections.

General instructions
1. Nurse should wash her hands before and after every eye treatment:
   a. To prevent spreading medication to her own eyes.
   b. To prevent spreading medication to eyes of other patients.
   c. To prevent danger of combining two unlike drugs — for example, spreading atropine from her hands to the eyes of a patient who is getting eserine.
   d. To prevent carrying infection to a patient's eyes or to her own.
2. Never *drop* the medication on the cornea.
3. Do not let the dropper touch the eye.
4. Never use a dropper more than once unless it has been properly cleaned and sterilized.

Solutions used
Eye drugs as ordered.

Temperature of solution
Room to body temperature.

Amount of solution used
1 or 2 drops.

Necessary articles
Small enamel container with cover for sterile droppers.
Small covered enamel container with sterile cotton balls.
Transfer forceps in antiseptic solution.
Medicine droppers, as many as needed.
Kidney basin for used cotton balls and droppers.
Small tray.

Preparation of equipment
1. Cover tray with clean towel.
2. Enamel containers, lifter, and container with antiseptic solution should be boiled daily and kept sterile in the Treatment Room.

3. Droppers that have been cleaned and boiled are replaced in the enamel container for that purpose.
4. Secure the medication ordered and place with the other articles on tray, or, if several medications are to be instilled, the eye medication tray may be carried with the tray. Carry tray to bedside.

Preparation of patient
1. Tell patient what the treatment is to be.
2. Have him turn his head in such a way that the eye in which drop is to be put is on the lower side, so that medication will not run into opposite eye or toward nose.

Procedure
1. With the transfer forceps secure a dropper from its container.
2. With the transfer forceps secure a cotton ball from its container.
3. Draw required amount of solution into dropper.
4. Pull down lower lid with index or middle finger, pressing firmly against the molar bone. Have patient look up.
5. Drop the medication at the inner or outer canthus of the eye. Touch the drop on the membrane of the lid before breaking it off from the dropper. The medicine must *run* into the eye, not drop.
6. Have patient close eyelids slowly to spread the drops. The eyelids should never be squeezed shut, for the medication will then be forced out of the eye. Catch the overflow of the medication with the cotton ball.
7. With the index finger exert pressure at the inner canthus over the opening into the tear sac in order to prevent drops from entering the nose. This is necessary for the following reason: Such drugs as atropine and cocaine are sometimes applied in solutions that are strong enough to produce poisonous symptoms in children or susceptible adults if they are absorbed.
8. With children who squeeze eyelids tightly when medication is to be instilled, hold the head in position while a drop of the medication is placed on the inner canthus of the eye. When the eye is opened, the medication will run into the eye. Otherwise carry out the procedure as given.

After-care of patient
1. Dry the eyelids and be sure the face is left clean and dry.
2. Leave patient as comfortable as possible.
3. Leave unit in order.

After-care of equipment
1. Empty used cotton balls into waste container.
2. Place used eye droppers in cold water and rinse thoroughly.

3. Wash in soap solution, separating bulb and glass.
4. Rinse in warm water and replace bulb on glass.
5. Boil for 5 minutes.
6. Replace in sterile container on tray.
7. Wash kidney basin in soap solution and replace on tray.

Record
1. In treatment and medication column: hour, kind, and quantity of solution instilled.
2. In nurse's remarks column: comfort or discomfort caused.
3. All charting is followed by nurse's initials.

References
Manhattan Eye, Ear, Nose, and Throat Hospital, *Nursing in Diseases of Eye, Ear, Nose, and Throat* (4th edition), p. 146.
Lewis, Eliason, Ferguson, *Surgical Nursing*, p. 352.

Administration of Eye Ointments

For eyelids
Squeeze a small amount of the ointment on the little finger and massage the eyelids.

For eye
1. Lower lid:
   a. Squeeze small amount into lower lid, close eye, and allow ointment to spread over conjunctiva.
2. Upper lid:
   a. Evert lid.
   b. Squeeze small amount of ointment from tube across cartilege portion and close eye gently. Allow to spread.

Administration of eye powders
1. Generally placed on upper lid of eye.
   a. Evert lid.
   b. Brush powder from sterile applicator lightly on everted lid. Close eyelids gently and allow powder to dissolve into moisture within eye.

Eye Irrigation

Purpose
1. To insure cleanliness.
2. To control infection.

General instructions
1. Where there is a copious discharge and Neisserian infection, the nurse should protect herself by wearing a gown and rubber gloves. The patient should be isolated and all contagious technique used.

2. If only one eye is to be treated, protect the other eye by using a Buller shield or some protective pad or dressing. The Buller shield is considered the best protection.

3. If both eyes are to be treated, a separate tray with separate equipment should be used for each eye, and the hands of the nurse should be scrubbed before the procedure, after the care of the first eye, and after the procedure.

4. Always direct the stream from the inner toward the outer canthus of the eye and dry the eyelids with a cotton pledget, wiping in one direction.

5. Never let the stream of solution flow from a height of more than 2 or 3 inches above the eye.

6. The cotton pledget used for wiping and cleaning the eyes must *never* be allowed to come in contact with the cornea. The slightest wisp of cotton may perforate an inflamed cornea.

7. Never exert pressure on the eyeball.

8. Never use force in opening the eyelids.

9. If instrument or eye dropper is used, never let the tip of the article touch the eye.

10. Be very sure that the percentage strength and temperature of the solution are accurate; the cornea is very sensitive and easily irritated.

11. Wash hands before and after treatment.

Solutions used
1. Boric acid solution 2–4 per cent.
2. Physiological saline solution.
3. Bichloride of mercury 1/10,000.
4. Potassium permanganate 1/5000; rarely used.

Temperature of solution
90°–95° F.

Amount of solution used
As much as is necessary to give desired result.

Necessary articles
Several large cotton balls.
Medicine dropper.
Asepto syringe, 2-ounce ear syringe, or irrigating can with rubber tubing and glass tip.
Container for solution ordered; use 6–8 ounce bottle if asepto syringe is used.
Kidney basin.
Face towel.
Rubber protector.
Flask of sterile solution.

Sterile towel.
Paper bag and safety pin.
Tray.
Cellu-cotton pad.

Preparation of equipment
1. Cover half of tray with sterile towel folded in half.
2. Fold back half of towel.
3. After boiling for 10 minutes place on towel:
   a. Container for solution.
   b. Kidney basin.
   c. Irrigating articles.
   Add sterile cotton balls. Cover articles with part of sterile towel that has been folded back.
4. In the dressing room heat solution to proper temperature by placing flask in a container of hot water. Test temperature with sterile thermometer.
5. Place warm solution, rubber protector, face towel, paper bag, and safety pin on unsterile half of tray.
6. Carry tray to bedside and place on bedside table.

Preparation of patient
1. Tell patient what the treatment is to be.
2. Screen patient, if in a ward; if in a room, place screen before door.
3. For greater convenience have patient move to edge of bed.
4. Remove all but one pillow from under patient's head.
5. Patient is to lie in a dorsal recumbent position with head tilted slightly back, chin well up, and head turned toward eye that is to be irrigated.

Procedure
1. Fold top of paper bag and fasten to bedside with safety pin.
2. Protect pillow and bedding with rubber protector covered with face towel and placed well under the head to the patient's neck.
3. Place kidney basin, protected by the cellu-cotton pad, close to face of patient, between the eye and the ear, to catch the flow of solution and prevent it from running down into the ear. Patient may assist in holding basin in place.
4. Wash off adherent discharge from lids with cotton balls moistened in the solution ordered, and discard used cotton balls into paper bag. Never put a used cotton ball back into the solution.
5. Saturate the large cotton ball with the solution ordered and slowly squeeze solution out in a small steady stream from the twisted tail of the cotton ball; direct stream from inner to

outer canthus of the eye. Medicine dropper or ear bulb can be used instead of cotton ball.

6. If unable to open the lids at first, irrigate over outside until lids can be separated.

7. Separate the lids by making traction with third and fourth fingers of left hand upon the flesh above and below lids, exerting all necessary pressure upon the frontal and molar bones, never on the eyeball. The thumb and index fingers are left free for grasping or holding in case of an emergency in which the right hand must be free.

8. When the eye has been thoroughly cleansed of all discharge, dry lids with cotton ball, wiping away from the eye.

After-care of patient

1. Be sure patient's face is clean and dry.
2. Leave patient as comfortable as possible.
3. See that unit is left in order.

After-care of equipment

1. If repeated irrigations are to be given the same patient, the tray may be left on lower shelf of bedside table between irrigations. Reboil and reset at least once daily and as often in addition as necessary.
2. Remove kidney basin, empty solution, wash with soap and water, boil, and replace on tray.
3. The flask containing the warmed solution should be taken to dressing room and kept there until it is necessary to reheat for the procedure.
4. Discard and replace paper bag as often as necessary.
5. If only one irrigation is ordered, the complete equipment is removed, cleaned, boiled for 5 minutes, and put away.

Record

1. In treatment and medication column: time, kind, strength, amount of solution used, results, discharge, etc.
2. In nurse's remarks column: comfort or discomfort caused.
3. Nurse's initials follow all charting.

References

Parkinson, *Diseases of the Eye, Ear, Nose, and Throat for Nurses*, p. 105.

Roberts, *Eye, Ear, Nose, and Throat Diseases for Nurses*, p. 55.

Application of Hot Compresses to the Eye

Purpose

1. To relieve pain.
2. To relieve inflammation and congestion.

3. To provide comfort for the patient.
4. To provide localized heat.

General instructions
1. If there is a discharge from the eye, it should be cleansed before hot applications are applied.
2. Any discharge from the eye should be considered infectious. Therefore the compresses should not be used again.
3. The compresses should be scrupulously clean and smooth.
4. The compresses should not extend over the nose nor eyebrow.
5. All applications should be made with a firm and sure but gentle touch.
6. Avoid pressure on the eyeball.
7. Avoid the use of forceps near the eyes; a sudden jerking of the patient's head may cause injury to the eye.
8. Unless ordered, do not apply heat for more than 20 minutes at a time; the blood vessels are completely dilated in that time if the procedure is properly carried out. Continued heat when the vessels are completely dilated may cause waterlogging and destruction of tissue. At least two hours should elapse between applications unless otherwise ordered.
9. When medications are to be instilled, they should follow the hot application.
10. The nurse's hands must be washed before and after the procedure.
11. When electric appliances are used, the cord and all connections should be carefully examined to prevent short-circuiting.
12. Avoid burning the patient, either with hot sponges or electric light or as a result of using faulty electric cords.

Solutions used
1. Boric acid solution.
2. Physiological salt solution.

Temperature of solution
120°–130° F.

Amount of solution used
As much as is necessary to keep compresses moist and hot, when electric bulb is used to supply heat, throughout the procedure.

Necessary articles
Olive oil in medicine glass.
Eye pad.
Gauze 4 inches square.
Two strips of ¼-inch adhesive 5 inches long.
Container for solution ordered.
Medicine dropper.

Cotton balls.
Kidney basin.
Face towel.
25-watt carbon electric bulb with wire guard; cord and connections.
Black stocking to cover guard.
Tray.

Preparation of equipment
1. Cover half of tray with sterile towel folded in half.
2. Fold back half of towel.
3. After boiling for 10 minutes, place on towel:
   a. Container for solution.
   b. Medicine dropper.
   c. Kidney basin.
   Add:
   d. Sterile eye pad.
   e. A few cotton balls.
   f. Compress 4 inches square.
4. Cover articles with part of sterile towel that has been folded back.
5. Heat solution to its proper temperature in the dressing room by placing flask in container of hot water. Test temperature with sterile thermometer.
6. Place solution, face towel, adhesive strips, olive oil, and electric equipment on unsterile half of tray.
7. Carry tray to bedside and place on bedside table.

Preparation of patient
1. Tell patient what treatment is to be.
2. Have patient move to side of bed and lie in dorsal recumbent position.
3. Remove all but 1 pillow from under the head.

Procedure
1. Attach electric-light extension. Test light before bringing bulb to patient's bedside.
2. Place face towel across chest.
3. If there is a discharge from the eye, moisten a cotton ball with the solution and cleanse the eye.
4. Dry with cotton ball.
5. Place sterile cotton eye pad over the eye and fasten with adhesive strips placed parallel to each other and to the nose.
6. With a cotton ball sparingly apply olive oil to the tissue surrounding the eye to prevent irritation and drying from the heat.

7. Moisten eye pad thoroughly by using medicine dropper and solution ordered.
8. Cover with sterile dry compress to provide thickness and protection.
9. Turn on the light and have patient hold it next to the compress, maintaining a steady heat, as hot as patient can bear comfortably.
10. Continue treatment for 20 minutes unless otherwise ordered.

After-care of patient
1. Remove and shut off light.
2. Remove and discard dressing and pad into kidney basin.
3. Dry eye with cotton ball.
4. Remove oil from face by wiping it off with cotton ball. Wash off if patient wishes. Leave the face dry and patient as comfortable as possible.
5. Leave unit in order.

After-care of equipment
1. Empty kidney basin. Wash with soap and water, boil, and replace on tray.
2. If repeated hot packs are ordered, tray may be left on bottom shelf of bedside table with enough equipment for several procedures.
3. The solution should be removed to dressing room and reheated for each procedure.
4. Reboil and reset tray at least once daily and as often in addition as necessary.

Record
1. In treatment and medication column: time, treatment, duration, amount of discharge.
2. In nurse's remarks column: comfort or discomfort caused by treatment.
3. Nurse's initials follow all charting.

Necessary articles when hot wet compresses are used to supply heat
Dressing bowl with solution as ordered.
6 sponges of folded gauze 4 inches square if eye is not discharging; more if compresses must be discarded every time.
Basin with hot water into which flask of sterile solution ordered can be placed, heated, and kept hot.
2 forceps.
Face towel.
Paper bag and safety pin.
Cotton balls.
Olive oil.
Tray.

Preparation of equipment
1. Cover half of tray with sterile towel folded in two.
2. Fold back half of towel.
3. After boiling for 10 minutes place on towel:
   a. Container for solution.
   b. 2 forceps.
   Add sterile cotton balls.
4. Cover articles with part of sterile towel that has been folded back.
5. Neatly arrange unsterile equipment on unsterile portion of tray.
6. Carry tray to bedside and place on bedside table.

Preparation of patient
1. Tell patient what treatment is to be.
2. Have patient move to side of bed and lie in dorsal recumbent position.
3. Remove all but 1 pillow from under the head.

Procedure
1. Fasten paper bag at side of bed with safety pin.
2. Place face towel across chest well under patient's chin.
3. With a cotton ball sparingly apply olive oil to the skin surrounding eye to avoid drying and irritation.
4. If there is a discharge from the eye, protect the well eye by using a Buller shield or gauze square to cover it.
5. Cleanse the discharge from the eye by moistening cotton ball in solution and gently wiping from the inner toward outer canthus. Avoid pressure on the eyeball and injury to the cornea.
6. Place sponges in container and pour hot solution over them.
7. Wring sponges fairly dry with forceps and apply with fingers, folding gauze to fit the eye (generally double the 4x4 sponge). Two sponges folded double form a good pack.
8. Cup the hand over the sponges to retain the heat as much as possible without pressure.
9. Change every 30–60 seconds, as necessary.
10. Discard soiled sponges into paper bag.
11. Change solution, and add to it as often as is necessary to maintain the proper temperature.

Note. — When an electric hot plate is used to keep solution hot, it should be placed on a separate bedside table behind the head of the bed, out of reach of the patient. All precautions should be taken into consideration in testing connections and cord. Avoid overheating solution and burning patient.

After-care of patient
1. Remove and discard dressing.
2. Dry eye with cotton ball.
3. Remove oil from face by wiping it off with cotton ball. Wash off if patient wishes. Leave face dry and patient as comfortable as possible.
4. Leave unit in order.

After-care of equipment
1. Same as previous procedure.

Record
1. In treatment and medication column: time, treatment, duration, amount of discharge.
2. In nurse's remarks column: comfort or discomfort caused by treatment.
3. Nurse's initials follow all charting.

References
Manhattan Eye, Ear, Nose, and Throat Hospital, *Nursing in Diseases of the Eye, Ear, Nose, and Throat*, pp. 132, 136, 137.
Lewis, Eliason, Ferguson, *Surgical Nursing*, pp. 354–55.

Application of Cold Compresses to the Eye

Purpose
1. To relieve inflammation and congestion.
2. To relieve pain.
3. To make patient comfortable.

General instructions
1. Make applications of compresses with a firm and sure but gentle touch.
2. Avoid pressure on the eyeball.
3. Be sure compresses are scrupulously clean and smooth.
4. Be sure compresses do not extend over nose or eyebrow.
5. Any discharge from the eyes should be considered infectious; therefore such compresses should not be applied more than once.
6. Treatment is not to be continued for more than 20 minutes unless otherwise ordered, and at least one hour should elapse between treatments.
7. The nurse's hands must be washed before and after the procedure.

Necessary articles
6 gauze sponges 4 inches square.
Dressing bowl for ice with gauze tied over the top to form a hammock for the sponges.

Face towel.
Cotton balls.
Boric acid solution.
Paper bag with safety pin if eye is draining, otherwise a kidney
basin.
Rubber binder or string.
Tray.

Preparation of equipment
1. Cover tray with clean towel.
2. Place an open sterile sponge over dressing bowl to form a
hammock, and use rubber band or string to fasten it under the
basin.
3. Place small block of ice on hammock.
4. Arrange equipment neatly on the tray and cover with clean
towel.
5. Carry tray to bedside and place on bedside table.

Preparation of patient
1. Tell patient what treatment is to be.
2. Have patient move to side of bed and lie in dorsal recumbent
position.
3. Remove all but one pillow from under head.

Procedure
1. Fasten paper bag to bedside.
2. Place towel across patient's chest well under chin.
3. If there is a discharge from the eye, cleanse with cotton ball
moistened with boric acid solution.
4. Fold compresses once, moisten with boric acid solution, and
place on ice.
5. When compresses are thoroughly chilled, place on eye, and
change every 15–30 seconds, as necessary, to keep them cold.
6. If there is drainage from the eye, the compress should not be
used again; drop into paper bag.

After-care of patient
1. Remove chest towel.
2. Dry the eye with cotton ball and the face with towel.
3. Leave patient comfortable.
4. Leave unit in order.

After-care of equipment
1. If repeated cold packs are ordered, the tray may be left on the
lower shelf of the bedside table between treatments. Refill ice
bowl at each treatment.
2. Empty paper bag or kidney basin as often as necessary and
replace.

Record
1. In treatment and medication column: time, treatment, and duration.
2. In nurse's remarks column: condition of eyes and effect of treatment.
3. Nurse's initials follow all charting.

References
Manhattan Eye, Ear, Nose, and Throat Hospital, *Nursing in Diseases of the Eye, Ear, Nose, and Throat*, pp. 132, 138, 139.
Lewis, Eliason, Ferguson, *Surgical Nursing*, p. 355.

Dry Treatment of Ears

Purpose
1. To insure continual drainage from running ear, thereby checking the infection and preventing it from spreading.
2. To prevent the accumulation, hardening, and blocking up of the discharge from a running ear.
3. To promote the comfort of patient.

General instructions
1. Be sure the size of the wick is only slightly smaller than the ear canal.
2. Be sure the wick is long enough to reach down to the ear drum, leaving a small tuft of cotton outside the canal so that the wick can be easily removed.
3. Remove the wick when it is two-thirds saturated with discharge and replace with a clean wick.

Necessary articles
Sterile cotton balls.
Applicators or toothpicks.
Paper bag and safety pin.
Tray.

Preparation of equipment
1. Prepare articles on tray, carry articles to bedside, and place on bedside table.

Preparation of patient
1. Tell patient what the treatment is to be.
2. Have patient move to edge of bed.
3. Remove all but 1 pillow under the head, and have the patient turn the affected ear up.

Procedure
1. Fasten paper bag to bedside with safety pin.
2. Make a thin, flat sheet of cotton 1 inch wide and $2\frac{1}{2}$ inches long from the cotton ball.

3. Place an applicator or the wide end of a toothpick in this sheet of cotton so that about ½ inch of cotton extends beyond the end of the applicator to prevent injuring the drum when inserting the wick.
4. Roll the sheet smoothly and evenly about the applicator or toothpick to the size of the canal.
5. Have a soft, loose fluff of cotton at the external end of the wick so that it may be easily grasped with the fingers and removed.
6. Secure a firm hold of the pinna and pull it upward and backward to straighten the canal, and insert the wick to the ear drum. Avoid exerting pressure on the ear drum.
7. Twist applicator backward one or two turns to loosen it from wick and remove applicator, leaving wick in the canal.
8. Remove wick when two-thirds moist with drainage, discard into paper bag, and insert a clean wick.
9. Be sure ear canal is properly cleaned before leaving wick in it.

After-care of patient
1. Keep external ear clean and dry at all times.
2. Keep bed linen free from ear discharge.
3. Make the patient as comfortable as possible.
4. Leave unit in order.

After-care of equipment
1. For a draining ear, leave tray on lower bedside shelf at all times.
2. Reset as often as necessary, but at least once daily.
3. Change paper bag whenever necessary.

Record
1. In treatment and medication column: time, treatment, duration, amount of drainage.
2. In nurse's remarks column: comfort or discomfort caused by treatment.
3. Nurse's initials follow all charting.

Ear Irrigation

Purpose
1. To cleanse the external ear.
2. To relieve inflammation and congestion.
3. To remove accumulated discharge from running ears.

General instructions
1. The flow should be gentle, steady, and continuous.
2. Air bubbles should not be forced into the canal.

3. A pointed instrument should never be put into the ear. Prevent injury to the canal by covering the irrigating tip with rubber tubing.
4. Never use a hot or cold solution in the ear, as it produces dizziness, pain, and discomfort.
5. Avoid pressure in the ear.
6. Report pain, dizziness, or any unusual complaint made by patient and stop procedure immediately when it is made.
7. Wash hands before and after procedure.

Solutions used
1. Weak sodium bicarbonate solution (1 level teaspoon to 1 quart, 1 dram to 1 quart).
2. Normal saline.
3. Tap water.

Amount of solution used
500 cc.

Temperature of solution
105° F. for cleansing.
110° F. to relieve pain and inflammation.

Necessary articles
Tray.
Irrigating can with tubing 2 feet long with stopcock.
Lucas ear irrigating tip with ½-inch rubber protector at the tip that is inserted into the ear.
Rubber protector.
Face towel.
Kidney basin.
Cotton balls for wicks.
Solution as ordered.
Applicators.
Standard.
Graduate for measuring solution.

Preparation of equipment
1. Boil irrigating can and tubing, tip, and kidney basin.
2. Place a clean towel on the tray.
3. Prepare the solution as ordered. Test with thermometer.
4. Close stopcock and pour solution into irrigating can.
5. Place 2 or 3 cotton balls and applicators on tray.
6. Cover rubber protector with face towel, fold, and place on tray.
7. Be sure that the Lucas irrigating tip is detached from tubing. Place in kidney basin.
8. Cover tray with clean towel and carry with standard to bedside. Place tray on bedside table.

Preparation of patient
1. Tell patient what the treatment is to be.
2. Screen completely, if in a ward; if in a room, place screen before door.
3. Patient may lie down in dorsal recumbent position or sit up in a chair.
4. Fold top bedding down once if patient is unable to sit up.
5. Place covered rubber protector well under head and over shoulder of patient.

Procedure
1. Hang irrigating can 10–12 inches above head of patient.
2. Place kidney basin under the ear and have the patient hold it in place if possible.
3. Open stopcock and expel air from tubing.
4. Irrigate the external ear gently.
5. Cleanse and dry external ear with cotton ball.
6. Attach Lucas ear irrigating tip to tubing and insert in the ear.
7. Hold external ear upward and backward to straighten the canal.
8. Open stopcock slowly until a steady, gentle stream is secured.
9. Continue until all of solution has been used.
10. Dry the ear canal thoroughly with cotton wicks or applicators and the external ear with cotton balls or towel.

After-care of patient
1. Remove rubber protector and fold back bed covers.
2. Be sure patient's face, ear, and neck are clean and dry.
3. Note appearance of patient and effect of treatment.
4. Leave unit in order.

After-care of equipment
1. Remove and replace screen and standard.
2. Carry tray to dressing room and wash irrigating can, Lucas irrigator, and kidney basin in soap solution and boil 5 minutes. *The tray should always be left clean.*
3. Replace all equipment on tray and see that it is ready for use before it is put away.

Record
1. In treatment and medication column: time, treatment, amount and kind of solution used, amount and kind of discharge.
2. In nurse's remarks column: comfort or discomfort caused by treatment.
3. Nurse's initials follow all charting.

References

Manhattan Eye, Ear, Nose, and Throat Hospital, *Nursing in Diseases of the Eye, Ear, Nose, and Throat,* 4th edition, p. 210.

Roberts, *Eye, Ear, Nose, and Throat Diseases for Nurses,* p. 69.

Mouth and Throat Irrigation

Purpose

1. To relieve inflammation and congestion.
2. To cleanse all parts of the mouth and throat.
3. To make the patient comfortable.

General instructions

1. When the throat irrigation is for the purpose of relieving inflammation and congestion, have solution as hot as patient can stand it, and continue the procedure until patient is relieved.
2. Be sure that all parts of throat are reached by moving irrigation tip from side to side of mouth.
3. By stopping the flow of the solution from time to time, allow patient to breathe and clear the throat.

Solutions used

1. Physiological salt solution.
2. Dobell's solution 50 per cent.
3. Sodium bicarbonate solution, 1 dram to 1 quart of water.
4. Magnesium sulphate solution, 1 dram to 1 quart of water.
5. Hydrogen peroxide solution 25 per cent.
6. Boric acid solution 2 per cent.
7. Potassium permanganate, 1/10,000.

Temperature of solution

105°–120° F. or as hot as patient can stand it.

Amount of solution used

1000 cc.

Necessary articles

Tray.

Quart-size irrigating can with tubing 2–3 feet long, stopcock, and glass connecting point with smaller tubing 2–3 inches long connected to glass point.

Tongue blade.

Rubber protector.

Cotton drawsheet to cover rubber protector.

Safety pin to fasten protector.

1000 cc. graduate for solution.

Hand basin for return flow.

Preparation of equipment
1. Be sure that stopcock on tubing is wide open.
2. Boil irrigating can, tubing, stopcock, glass point, narrower tubing, and 1000 cc. graduate for 10 minutes.
3. Prepare solution in 1000 cc. graduate. Tap water may be used for these solutions. Use clean thermometer for testing temperature.
4. Close stopcock on tubing before pouring solution into irrigating can.
5. Cover rubber protector with drawsheet and fold neatly.
6. Cover tray with clean towel, carry to bedside, and place on bedside table.

Preparation of patient
1. Tell patient what the treatment is to be.
2. Screen patient completely, if in a ward; if in a room, place screen before door.
3. Place patient in position:
   a. Prone or semi-recumbent, near edge of bed, with head turned to one side.
   b. Sitting up in bed or in a chair.

Procedure with patient in semi-recumbent or prone position
1. Place covered rubber protector under head and over shoulder and chest.
2. Place hand basin where it will catch return flow.
3. Expel air from tubing.
4. With right hand hold glass point and tubing on tongue blade and insert into patient's mouth. The tongue blade is used to depress the tongue, while the point may be moved about — the narrow, soft rubber tubing extending beyond the end of tongue blade.
5. By pressing down on back part of tongue with tongue blade, prevent the tubing from touching the back part of throat and causing patient to gag and cough. With left hand open the stopcock and slowly elevate the irrigating can until a steady stream of solution is secured.
6. Make sure that the stream reaches all parts of the throat by moving the glass point on the blade without moving the tongue blade.

Procedure with patient sitting up in bed or in a chair
1. Adjust rubber sheet about neck of patient and pin with safety pin.
2. Place hand basin in patient's lap.
3. Have patient lower head over basin and irrigate his throat

himself. A tongue blade is not necessary unless the patient prefers to use it.

4. Stay with patient and make sure that he rotates the tip of the irrigating point so that all parts of the throat are reached.
5. Place articles on tray and remove to dressing room.

After-care of patient
1. Remove rubber protector and covering and place on tray.
2. Cleanse face and dry.
3. Leave patient comfortable.
4. Leave unit in order.

After-care of equipment
1. Empty hand basin into hopper and wash with soap solution.
2. Wash irrigating can, connecting point and tubing, and 1000 cc. graduate in soap solution; boil for 5 minutes and replace on tray, if tray is to be used again; otherwise replace on shelf. *Note.* — When repeated irrigations are to be given the same patient, a tray may be kept set up for that purpose in the dressing room. Label tray with name of patient and kind of tray. In this instance it is not necessary to boil the irrigating can every time the procedure is done. Disconnect the glass point and narrow tubing, wash in soap solution, and boil after each procedure.

Record
1. In treatment and medication column: time, treatment, amount, and kind of solution used.
2. In nurse's remarks column: comfort or discomfort caused by treatment.
3. Nurse's initials follow all charting.

References
Harmer, *Principles and Practice of Nursing,* pp. 791–95.

Nasal Irrigation

Purpose
1. To soften and remove discharges.
2. To relieve congestion, swelling, and pain.

General instructions
1. Have irrigating can 3 inches above patient to prevent washing the discharge into Eustachian tube.
2. Instruct patient to breathe through the mouth. Be sure that mouth is kept wide open.
3. Do not allow patient to blow his nose nor attempt to swallow while nose is filled with solution.
4. Never place a glass tube in the nostril.

Solutions usually ordered
1. Physiological salt solution.
2. Boric acid solution.
3. Sodium bicarbonate solution.

Temperature of solution
1. 105°–115° F.

Position of patient
1. Sitting in a chair with head flexed on the chest.
2. Dorsal recumbent position, with head turned to side and nostril into which the tip is to be inserted uppermost.

Necessary articles
Tray.
Quart-size irrigating can with tubing 2–3 feet long, stopcock, and glass connection point with smaller tubing 2–3 inches long connected to glass point.
Rubber protector.
Cotton drawsheet to cover rubber protector.
Safety pin to fasten protector.
1000 cc. graduate to prepare solution.
Hand basin for return flow.

Preparation of equipment
1. Be sure that stopcock on tubing is wide open.
2. Boil irrigating can, tubing, stopcock, glass point, narrower tubing, and 1000 cc. graduate for 10 minutes.
3. Prepare the solution in the 1000 cc. graduate. Tap water may be used for these solutions. Use clean thermometer for testing temperature.
4. Close stopcock on tubing before pouring solution into irrigating can.
5. Cover rubber protector with drawsheet and fold neatly.
6. Cover tray with clean towel, carry to bedside and place on bedside table.

Preparation of patient
1. Tell patient what the treatment is to be.
2. Screen patient completely, if in a ward; if in a room, place screen before door.
3. Place patient in position:
   a. Prone or semi-recumbent, near edge of bed.
   b. Sitting up in bed or in a chair.

Procedure
1. Place covered rubber protector under the head, covering shoulder and chest.
2. Place hand basin where it will catch the return flow.

3. Expel the air from the tubing.
4. Gently raise the tip of the nostril and insert the rubber tip into the nostril and start flow, rather slowly at first, then at slightly increased rate.
5. The solution should return through the opposite nostril and the mouth.
6. Continue the treatment until satisfied with results, or until desired amount has been given.
7. Place articles on tray and remove to dressing room.

After-care of patient
1. Remove rubber protector and covering and place on tray.
2. Cleanse face and dry.
3. Have patient wait at least 3 minutes before blowing the nose, when he should blow both sides at once.

After-care of equipment
1. Empty hand basin into hopper and wash with soap solution.
2. Wash irrigating can, connecting point, tubing, and graduate with soap solution.
3. Boil for 5 minutes all material used.
4. Replace on tray if treatment is to be given again; otherwise replace on shelf.
   (See note concerning routine throat irrigations.)

Record
1. In treatment and medication column: time, treatment, amount and kind of solution, discharge.
2. In nurse's remarks column: comfort or discomfort caused, dyspnea relieved.
3. Nurse's initials follow all charting.

References
Harmer, *Principles and Practice of Nursing*, pp. 795–96.

Administration of Nose Drops

Purpose
1. To combat and prevent spread of infection.
2. To contract congested nasal mucosa, thus relieving dyspnea and discomfort.
3. To lessen coryzal secretions.

Solutions used
1. To contract membranes: nasal oils.
2. As disinfectants: neosilvol, argyrol.

General instructions
1. The position of the head rather than the force with which the

drop is given determines how much of the mucosa will be affected by the medication.

2. It is not necessary to use a large quantity of the medication; 3 drops is the maximum.

Necessary articles
Tray.
Kidney basin.
Washed gauze.
Medication ordered.
Medicine dropper in sponge.

Preparation of equipment
1. Place articles on tray.
2. Carry to patient's bed.

Preparation of patient
1. Tell patient what the treatment is to be.
2. If an up patient have him lie across the bed with his head over the edge and lower than the bed.
3. If a bed patient, remove pillows from under head, place one pillow under shoulders so that head is lower than shoulders.

Procedure
1. Draw medicine dropper one-fourth full of the medication.
2. Gently raise tip of nostril, insert end of dropper just into end of nose, and squeeze medication out of dropper.
3. Have patient remain in this position until the medication reaches the throat. This will take from 2 to 3 minutes.
4. Let patient expectorate surplus medication into kidney basin.
5. After several minutes the patient may blow his nose if he desires.
6. Remove tray to dressing room.

After-care of patient
1. If a bed patient, replace pillows and make comfortable.

After-care of equipment
1. Wash and boil kidney basin and replace on shelf.
2. Remove bulb, clean glass part of medicine dropper with cotton applicator and soap and water; boil 5 minutes. Droppers used for nose drops should never be used for eye drops.

Record
1. In treatment and medication column: time, medication, strength, whether given in one or both nostrils.
2. In nurse's remarks column: relief or discomfort resulting from medication.
3. Nurse's initials follow all charting.

III. PREPARATION OF PATIENT FOR OPERATION

Minute details of pre-operative preparation vary in different hospitals, but the following are, for the most part, directions usually accepted.

General external preparation
1. Cleansing tub bath before putting into clean bed if patient is able to take tub bath; if unable to take tub bath, patient must have, at discretion of head nurse, thoroughly cleansing bed bath.
2. Inspect head for vermin, without patient's knowledge.
3. Trim and clean patient's finger- and toenails.
4. Pay special attention to umbilicus; this is most important.
5. Send specimen of urine to laboratory; get as soon as possible after admission.

Local preparation of operative area
1. Shave entire region, always allowing generous margin. Shave closely and carefully over entire region. Scrub with water and soap, using warm water. Rinse and dry.
2. Use clean gauze or cotton for washing. This should be done twelve hours before operation, if possible.
3. If emergency operation, omit soap and water and give dry shave. Further preparation is done in operating room.

Internal preparation
1. Day before operation nutritious food with little residue. The intestines should be empty.
2. Light tray for supper night before unless otherwise ordered.
3. Water up to but none after midnight.
4. No breakfast.
5. Enema, if ordered, before 7 A. M. on morning of operation; always report if effectual or not.
6. Douches as ordered for perineal cases before operation. Apply perineal pad after douche and fasten with T-binder.

Final preparation of patients
1. Patient must be ready half hour before time scheduled for Operating Room.
2. Comb and braid hair in two braids, tie ends with gauze or fasten with rubber bands ready to apply triangular bandage when brought with cart from operating room. Hairpins must never be left in.
3. Remove all jewelry and give to head nurse. Wedding ring

may be worn at discretion of head nurse, but must be tied to wrist with tape or gauze.

4. Put on clean gown, with opening at back; leave untied. Put on ether stockings, fasten with rubber band. No pins to be used in any way on patient.

5. Have patient empty bladder just before completing final preparation. Measure urine, and chart amount and time of voiding in red ink. Patient is catheterized only on doctor's order.

6. Hypodermic is given before going to operating room, according to order.

Preparation of specific areas for various operations

1. Abdominal operation:
   a. Shave from breasts to low on pubes and 4–5 inches on either side of median line. Scrub from breasts to pubes and to midline on either side. Give special attention to umbilicus.

2. Stomach:
   a. Shave from breast to below umbilicus and 4–5 inches on either side of median line. Scrub from breasts to pubes and to bed line on either side.

3. Kidney:
   a. Shave and scrub from sternum to the spine on the affected side and from axilla to the hip.

4. Breast:
   a. Shave axilla, chest on affected side, and upper arm. Scrub from hairline and ear to waistline, from nipple on opposite side to behind shoulder on the affected side, including upper arm.

5. Neck:
   a. Shave from hairline to nipple, axilla, and shoulder on affected side. Scrub from hairline to below nipple, axilla, shoulder, and upper arm.

6. Scalp:
   a. Order usually given by surgeon as to extent of surface to be prepared. It is an offense to shave a larger area than necessary. Therefore, to protect hospital and insure safe preparation of patient, the order must be written, if there are no written routine orders for the ward.

7. Leg or arm:
   a. Shave and prepare well above and below the affected parts.

8. Special operations (eye, ear, nose, throat, skin graft, etc.):
   a. Preparation varies with condition and operation. Routine

orders usually written for use of ward. If not, then order must be written for each patient.

9. Vaginal and rectal operations:
   a. Place the patient in dorsal position. Shave pubes and skin surrounding vulva and anus. Scrub lower abdomen, upper third of thighs, and inner surfaces of thighs and buttocks. Male patients should be prepared by the floor orderly or be prepared in the operating room.

References

Harmer, *Principles and Practice of Nursing*, pp. 326–32.

IV. STERILE SUPPLIES AND TRAYS

Purpose
1. To handle supplies with aseptic technique, that is, to prepare and handle them in such a manner as to prevent their carrying infection.

General instructions
1. Sterilized articles should never come in contact with unsterile articles. Should an article be contaminated, it must be resterilized before using.
2. Forceps for handling sterilized materials should be cleansed, boiled, and placed in a sterile jar containing fresh antiseptic solution. This must be done daily. If they are contaminated in any way, they must be boiled before being put back in the bottle. Avoid touching the top of the bottle when removing forceps.
3. Never allow any unsterile article (including hands and arms) to pass over any sterile material.
4. In removing sterile articles from a cover, remove the pins carefully. Never touch the inside of the cover. The contents may be removed by forceps into a sterile basin or may be dropped with forceps upon a sterile field.
5. In setting up a sterile tray, towels to cover the tray may be removed with forceps from the sterile package by picking them up carefully by the uppermost corner and placing over tray. Always have a double thickness of towel over a tray on which wet articles are to be placed.
6. In holding a sterile basin always hold by pressing the hands on the sides or by placing hands beneath the bottom of basin; never grasp it with fingers over the rim.
7. Sterile supply jars: lift the lid straight up from the jar and remove contents with forceps. If necessary to put lid down, place with the bottom side up, so that the inner rim will not come in contact with any unsterile thing. In replacing lid, avoid striking it against sides of jar.
8. Sterile pitchers: keep covered with sterile towels or sterile cover.
9. Pouring solutions:
   a. Remove stopper from bottles without unsterilizing bottom of cork.
   b. Clean mouth of bottle with antiseptic solution on sponge, then grasp the bottle, label side toward palm, and pour solution.

c. If no antiseptic is available, a small amount of solution may be poured from the mouth of the bottle to cleanse the bottle, holding over a sink or basin, never over the floor.

10. Be sure articles are clean before they are sterilized.

11. Wrap all articles before boiling to prevent breakage and the deposit of calcium salts on the articles.

12. Care of the patient:
   a. Expose only the part involved in the treatment.
   b. Keep patient warm and protected from draft.
   c. Protect the bedding from body fluid or medications used.
   d. Have patient in the most comfortable and convenient position for the treatment.

Preparation of Trays and Care of Articles Used

To sterilize articles used in the various procedures

1. Tubing, stopcocks, glasses, mixing bottles, beakers, pipettes, stirring rods, syringes, medicine droppers, small basins, etc.: sterilize by boiling 20 minutes.

2. Needles: sterilize by boiling 5 minutes or according to hospital routine.

3. Applicators, pledgets, small squares, and towels: keep sterile in covered jars in which they have been sterilized in autoclave.

4. Lifting forceps: keep sterile in antiseptic solution.

To set up sterile tray

1. Lift sterile towel with lifting forceps and spread over tray. The edge of the tray must be completely covered. Use second towel, if first towel is not large enough for this. If two towels are used, they must overlap and not just meet.

2. With lifting forceps, place sterilized articles on tray.

3. Cover with a sterile towel and carry to bedside.

To set up a tray a part of which is sterile

1. Lift sterile towel with lifting forceps, open, and spread over half of tray. Turn towel so that closed end is toward unsterile articles.

2. With lifting forceps place sterilized articles on sterile part of tray.

3. Cover with a sterile towel.

4. Arrange unsterile articles on tray.

Care of tubing and stopcocks

1. After using, drop immediately into cold water. As soon as possible rinse thoroughly by forcing water through with a syringe. Use a small brush for cleaning stopcocks.

2. Boil in water 3 minutes.

3. Rinse in cold water and dry the tubing by stripping. Complete the drying by forcing air through with a rubber bulb.

Care of needles
1. Following use, wash immediately in cold water. Boil 3 minutes.
2. Test for sharpness and hooks. Polish from base to point.
3. Dip stilette in polish, insert in the needle, and draw back and forth several times to polish caliber of needle. Force water through with bulb.
4. Dry the needles thoroughly.
5. Fill the syringe with alcohol 70 per cent and expel through the needle several times.
6. With rubber bulb blow out every drop of fluid. When perfectly dry, replace the wire, which has been dipped into liquid albolene.
7. Rub outside of needle with oiled cloth.
8. Place in a properly labeled container.

Venipuncture

Purpose
1. To withdraw blood from the circulation for diagnostic or therapeutic purposes.

Necessary articles
Skin preparation tray with:
Kidney basin.
Container of sterile toothpick applicators.
Forceps jar with lifting forceps in antiseptic solution.
Rubber protector with hand towel.
Wide-mouthed bottle with iodine.
Wide-mouthed bottle with alcohol.
Tourniquet.
Kidney basin for waste.
In addition:
Sterile package of 20 cc. syringe and intravenous needle 17x1½ or 19x1½.
Enamel cup with cold water for needle and syringe.
Container with cotton in bottom containing test tubes.

Preparation of equipment
1. Prepare the above-listed articles on tray.
2. Carry tray to bedside.

Preparation of the patient
1. Tell patient what treatment is to be.
2. Screen completely, if in a ward; if in a room, place screen before door.

3. Expose the arm by folding sleeve of gown away from field of treatment close to patient's body.
4. Place covered rubber protector under arm.
5. Place tourniquet under arm about 3 inches above elbow.
6. Sterilize the skin at the point of insertion of the needle (an area about 4 inches in radius) by cleansing with applicator dipped in iodine and then with alcohol. (The doctor usually does this.)
7. Just before the doctor is ready to start the treatment, open up syringe and needle.
8. Fasten tourniquet as tightly as is necessary to make the vein stand out prominently, and in such a way that the ends of tourniquet are pointed toward patient's shoulder.

Procedure
1. The doctor picks up the syringe and attaches the needle and inserts it into the vein. The nurse releases the tourniquet to allow the blood to flow freely. She must release it gently so as not to jar the needle out of the vein.
2. When the required amount of blood is obtained, the needle is withdrawn and pressure with a sponge is applied over the site of puncture. Have patient flex arm tightly.
3. Wash needle at once by drawing water into syringe and forcing through needle. Disconnect needle from syringe and place in water.

After-care of patient
1. Check to see that there is no bleeding from the puncture wound.
2. See that there are no blood stains on the patient or on his bedding.
3. Replace gown.
4. Remove screen and other articles and leave unit in order.
5. Keep patient warm and protected from drafts.

After-care of equipment
1. Rinse needles and syringe in cold water to remove the blood before it clots.
2. Wash and boil needles, syringe, glass, and forceps 3 minutes before you put them away, as previously instructed.

Record
1. Beside the order in the doctor's order book, indicate in red ink, when the tray is ready: "Tray set up" and initials.
2. When the treatment has been given, check the order with red ink and indicate the time in the margin.
3. In the treatment column: time, treatment, amount withdrawn, doctor, and nurse's initials.

4. In nurse's remarks column: any unusual symptom or reaction of the patient.

References
Kelley, *Textbook of Nursing Technique*, pp. 184–85.

Intravenous Injection of Typhoid Vaccine

Purpose
1. To introduce a foreign protein and thus stimulate production of antibodies.

Solutions used
1. Flask of physiological salt solution.
2. Typhoid vaccine.

Temperature of solution
1. Heat flask of salt solution to body temperature (110°–115° F.) by putting it in a basin of warm water 140° F.
2. Test temperature of solution by pouring it over your wrist.

Necessary articles
Tray.
Sterile articles:
3 cotton balls.
Towel.
2 venipuncture needles.
20 cc. syringe.
2 medicine glasses.
Tuberculin syringe.
Kidney basin.
Unsterile articles:
Small rubber sheet with towel.
Tourniquet.
Enamel basin with cold water.

Preparation of equipment
1. Prepare above-listed articles on tray.
2. Carry tray to bedside.

Preparation of patient
1. Tell patient what the treatment is to be.
2. Screen completely, if in a ward; if in a room, place screen before door.
3. Expose the arm by folding sleeve of gown away from field of treatment close to patient's body.
4. Place covered rubber protector under arm.
5. Place tourniquet under arm about 3 inches above elbow.
6. Sterilize the skin at the point of insertion of the needle (area

about 4 inches in radius) by cleansing with applicator dipped in iodine and then with alcohol. (The doctor usually does this.)
7. Just before the doctor is ready to start the treatment, open up syringe and needle.
8. Fasten tourniquet as tightly as is necessary to make the vein stand out prominently, and in such a way that the ends of tourniquet are pointed toward patient's shoulder.

Procedure
1. At bedside of patient the doctor prepares the vaccine and the physiological salt solution in a medicine glass, and draws the prepared solution into the syringe ready for use.
2. The tourniquet is applied until the needle is in the vein, when it is carefully released and the vaccine is slowly injected.
3. Typhoid vaccine is most frequently given subcutaneously. The technique is the same as that of any hypodermic injection.

After-care of patient
1. Check to see that there is no bleeding from the puncture wound.
2. See that there are no blood stains on the patient or on his bedding.
3. Replace gown.
4. Remove screen and other articles and leave unit in order.
5. Keep patient warm and protected from drafts.
6. Observe patient closely for change in pulse and respiration, and watch for chills, noting their duration and severity.
7. Apply external heat for chill.
8. Give oral fluids unless contra-indicated.
9. Take and record T. P. R. 30 minutes after the chill or as ordered.

After-care of equipment
1. Rinse needles and syringe in cold water to remove the blood before it clots.
2. Wash and boil needles, syringe, glass, and forceps 3 minutes before you put them away, as previously instructed.

Record
1. In order book check tray and procedure as for venepuncture.
2. In treatment and medication column: time, vaccine, amount, doctor, initials of nurse.
3. In nurse's remarks column: record symptoms and reaction of patient.
4. On temperature sheet: any rise in temperature with chill, as for any other chill. Often a separate temperature sheet is made out when this treatment is given.

References
Kelley, *Textbook of Nursing Technique*, p. 124.

Phenolsulphonephthalein Test

Purpose
1. To aid in the administration of the P. S. P. test so that the results will be as accurate and reliable as possible. Phenolsulphonephthalein is a dye which when injected into the body tissues is excreted by the kidneys. By injecting a definite amount and estimating the amount excreted within a certain time, the function of the kidneys is tested.

Necessary articles
Skin preparation tray with:
Kidney basin.
Container of sterile toothpick applicators.
Forceps jar with lifting forceps in antiseptic solution.
Rubber protector with hand towel.
Wide-mouthed bottle with iodine.
Wide-mouthed bottle with alcohol.
Tourniquet.
Kidney basin for waste.
In addition:
2 intravenous needles (usually 22x1½ inch) in tubes.
Sterile tuberculin syringe wrapped in sterile towel.
Ampule of dye.
File.

Preparation of equipment
1. Arrange articles on tray and carry to bedside.
2. Top of vial is cleaned with alcohol just before it is filed off.

Preparation of patient
1. Have patient empty bladder immediately before injection. This specimen is saved and used as the "control specimen."
2. Expose the arm by folding sleeve of gown away from field of treatment close to patient's body.
3. Place covered rubber protector under arm.
4. Place tourniquet under arm about 3 inches above elbow.
5. Sterilize the skin at the point of insertion of the needle (an area about 4 inches in radius) by cleansing with applicator dipped in iodine and then with alcohol. (The doctor usually does this.)
6. Just before the doctor is ready to start the treatment, unwrap syringe and needle.
7. Fasten tourniquet as tightly as is necessary to make the vein

stand out prominently, and in such a way that the ends of tourniquet are pointed toward patient's shoulder.

Procedure
1. Apply tourniquet until the needle is in the vein, release tourniquet.
2. The doctor injects the contents of the ampule of dye, which is 1 cc. of a salt solution containing 6 mg. of the dye.
3. Have patient drink 2 glasses of water just after the injection so that he will be able to void at the proper time.
4. If some other test is being given patient at the same time, the water may not be given. The nurse in charge will be of assistance to you in such event.
5. Collect urine at exactly 1 hour and at 2 hours after the injection, in separate bottles, and label. State on request blank the time of injection and time of voiding. If patient is unable to void, she must be catheterized. The doctor will usually write the order ahead of time.
6. Any medication and liquid nourishment that has been ordered may be given at the stated time, but solid food, such as daily trays, should be withheld until the last urination.

After-care of patient
1. Check to see that there is no bleeding from the puncture wound.
2. See that there are no blood stains on the patient or on his bedding.
3. Replace gown.
4. Remove screen and other articles and leave unit in order.
5. Keep patient warm and protected from drafts.

After-care of equipment
1. Rinse needles and syringe in cold water to remove the blood before it clots.
2. Wash and boil needles, syringe, glass, and forceps 3 minutes before you put them away, as previously instructed.

Record
1. In order book: check with red ink "Tray set up."
2. In treatment and medication column: hour, treatment, means of administering, doctor, nurse's initials. Time, amount in each specimen, specimen to laboratory.

Note. — When a dilution-concentration test is given the 2 glasses of water are not given at the time dye is injected. The patient has previously had water. When collecting a specimen from a patient who is having a P. S. P. and a dilution-concentration test done at one time, the urine is not sent to the laboratory until after specific gravity has been read. If the doctor catheterizes a male patient, he will ask for boric acid solution. Supply him with a 500 cc. graduate to measure accurately the amount of boric acid used.

Administration of Neosalvarsan

Purpose
1. To aid in introducing the medication, aseptically, into the vein, in treatment of syphilis.

Solution used
Flask of sterile, freshly distilled water.

Temperature of solution
78°–84° F. (room temperature).

Necessary articles
Sterile tray with:
20 cc. syringe.
2 intravenous needles, 22x1½ inch.
Medicine glass.
Skin preparation tray with:
Kidney basin.
Container of sterile toothpick applicators.
Forceps jar with lifting forceps in antiseptic solution.
Rubber protector with hand towel.
Wide-mouthed bottle with iodine.
Wide-mouthed bottle with alcohol.
Tourniquet.
Kidney basin for waste.
Flask of sterile distilled water.
Vial of salvarsan.

Preparation of equipment
1. Set up sterile tray as in previous procedures.
2. Carry both trays to bedside.

Preparation of patient
1. Roll up sleeve of gown, place rubber protector under arm.
2. Put on tourniquet as in venipuncture.

Procedure
1. When the doctor is about to begin his treatment, pour about 15 cc. of the sterile distilled water into the empty medicine glass.
2. Fill ampule containing powdered neosalvarsan and add powder slowly to the water. Usually the powder will dissolve without stirring if added slowly.
3. If mixing is necessary, draw solution into the syringe and carefully force it out. Keep end of syringe under solution

while mixing to avoid incorporating air into the solution. Oxygen causes a chemical change in the neosalvarsan which gives toxic symptoms in the patient.
4. The medication is given intravenously.
5. As soon as needle is in the vein, the tourniquet should be gently loosened.

After-care of patient
1. When needle is withdrawn, use pressure over puncture and have patient flex arm tightly. He should lie in recumbent position for at least 2 hours after the injection.
2. Watch for dizziness, nausea, ringing in ears, malaria chills.
3. If patient complains of local pain around puncture, it indicates that some of the solution is in the tissue. The doctor should be notified; local heat is usually ordered.

After-care of equipment
1. Rinse needles and syringe in cold water to remove the blood before it clots.
2. Wash and boil needles, syringe, glass, and forceps 3 minutes before you put them away, as previously instructed.

Record
1. In treatment and medication column: hour, medication, means of administering, doctor, nurse's initials.
2. In nurse's remarks column: reaction of patient to treatment.

References
Harmer, *Principles and Practice of Nursing,* pp. 506–07.
Kelley, *Textbook of Nursing Technique,* pp. 294–96.

Hypodermoclysis

Purpose
1. To supply fluid to the tissues subcutaneously in hemorrhage.
2. To stimulate the circulation in shock or collapse.
3. To restore body fluid lost during operation.
4. To dilute the poisons, flush the kidneys, and carry away the poisons in toxemia.

General instructions
1. Read label on flask when you get it from the Sterile Supply Room and again before you use it. Be sure you have the correct solution. Mistakes have occurred, and they are serious.
2. Carry out aseptic technique very strictly.

Temperature of solution
1. 120° F.

Amount of solution
  1. 500–2500 cc.

Site of injection
  1. Beneath skin of abdomen.
  2. In loose tissue at base of breasts.
  3. In thighs or buttocks.
  4. In the axillary line.

Solutions used
  1. Physiological salt solution contains sodium chloride 0.9 per cent.
  2. Locke's solution contains sodium chloride, potassium chloride, calcium chloride, sodium bicarbonate, and dextrose in amounts approximating that found in the plasma.
  3. Hartman's solution contains lactic acid, sodium chloride, potassium chloride, and calcium chloride in amounts approximating that found in blood plasma and kept neutral with carbonate free sodium hydroxide.

METHOD No. 1

Necessary articles
  Autoclaved tray from Sterile Supply Room with:
  Kelly flask with tubing and Y-glass tube extending from which are 2 tubings with adaptors on ends.
  Kidney basin.
  Medicine glass.
  Hemostat.
  3 sponges 3x3 inches.
  Sterile towel.
  2 hypodermic needles in tubes.
  2 hypodermoclysis needles 22x3 inches in tubes.
  Sterile wrapped 2 cc. syringe.
  Skin preparation tray with:
  Container of sterile toothpick applicators.
  Forceps jar with lifting forceps in antiseptic solution.
  Wide-mouthed bottle with iodine 3.5 per cent.
  Wide-mouthed bottle with alcohol 70 per cent.
  Adhesive ½ inch wide.
  Collodion.
  Flask of solution to be given.
  Flask of novocaine 1 per cent.
  Kidney basin.
  Standard.
  Hot-water bottle 120° F. (uncovered).
  Bath towel.

Preparation of equipment
1. Heat solution by setting in basin of water 140° F.
2. Take pins out of tray, but do not uncover.
3. Carry all equipment to bedside.

Preparation of patient
1. Screen completely and explain what the treatment is to be. Reassure patient if he is apprehensive of danger and pain.
2. If thighs are to be used for the injection, fold upper covers from just below area to foot of bed. Cover chest and abdomen with bath blanket and another heavy blanket if weather warrants. Place bath towel over pubic region and between legs.
3. If area below breasts is to be used, fold bedding down to below breasts, pin gown up, and cover chest with folded bath blanket.
4. A rubber-covered pillow placed under the knees helps to alleviate discomfort if injection is given in thighs.

Procedure
1. The areas for injection are prepared by the doctor, using sterile applicators and iodine 3.5 per cent and alcohol 70 per cent. One sterile towel is placed over edge of lower bedclothes.
2. Nurse opens tray and places on it syringe and needles.
3. Pour into medicine glass the amount of novocaine ordered. The doctor injects a small amount subcutaneously with the small hypodermic, and the rest is poured into the flask after the solution has been poured into it.
4. The doctor connects needles to tubing and holds Kelly flask while the nurse pours the solution into it. (See that clamps are closed first.)
5. Place sterile sponge in flask as a stopper.
6. Help doctor expel the air out of tubing before hanging up flask on standard.
7. The doctor puts each needle through a gauze square; the nurse holds one while he injects the other.
8. A 6-inch strip of adhesive is wound around hilt of needle and fastened to skin on each side. This holds the needles in place and also the gauze square.
9. The flow should be slow enough not to cause engorgement.
10. Place hot-water bottle around tube and cover with bath towel.
11. Be sure that patient is well covered and unit is neat.

After-care of patient
1. Watch for edema; if it occurs, make flow slower or shut it off for a time.

2. Watch patient's color and pulse closely.
3. To add solution to flask:
    a. Heat solution as previously.
    b. Remove sponge from flask and add desired amount of fluid, being sure to replace stopper. Do not wait until flask is empty before replenishing with fluid, for air would get into tubing.
4. Refill hot-water bottle every 30 minutes.
5. To discontinue the treatment:
    a. Screen patient.
    b. Shut off flow.
    c. Loosen adhesive tape and remove needles.
    d. Seal punctures with drop of collodion on small fluff of cotton.
    e. Place flask and tubing on tray.
    f. Remove blankets and replace covers neatly.
    g. Remove screen and extra equipment and leave unit neat and in order.

After-care of equipment
1. Remove trays from bedside table as soon as treatment has been started.
2. When treatment is finished, clean all articles and replace on tray from Sterile Supply Room.
3. Return it to Sterile Supply Room.
4. Station equipment is cleaned and put away in good condition.

Record
1. When tray is ready, write in red ink beside the order in doctor's order book, "Tray set up," with initials.
2. When treatment is finished, check order in margin with red ink, indicating the time.
3. In treatment and medication column: time, amount, kind of solution, novocaine added, treatment, by whom started. Time, amount, kind of solution added. Time, total amount, kind of solution taken, when discontinued.
4. In nurse's remarks column: any reaction of the patient, discomfort, etc.
5. On graphic sheet: total amount taken, in space opposite "subcutaneous."

METHOD No. 2

Necessary articles
Autoclaved tray from Sterile Supply Room with:
2-holed rubber stopper with 9¼-inch glass tubing through one hole and an L glass tube through the other. To this is at-

tached a piece of rubber tubing with Y tube and 2 pieces of
rubber tubing with adaptors (see diagram).
Metal clamp to fit over neck of flask.
Kidney basin.
Medicine glass.
Hemostat.
3 sponges 3x3 inches.
Sterile towel.
Other articles as in method no. 1.
Ring clamp for standard.

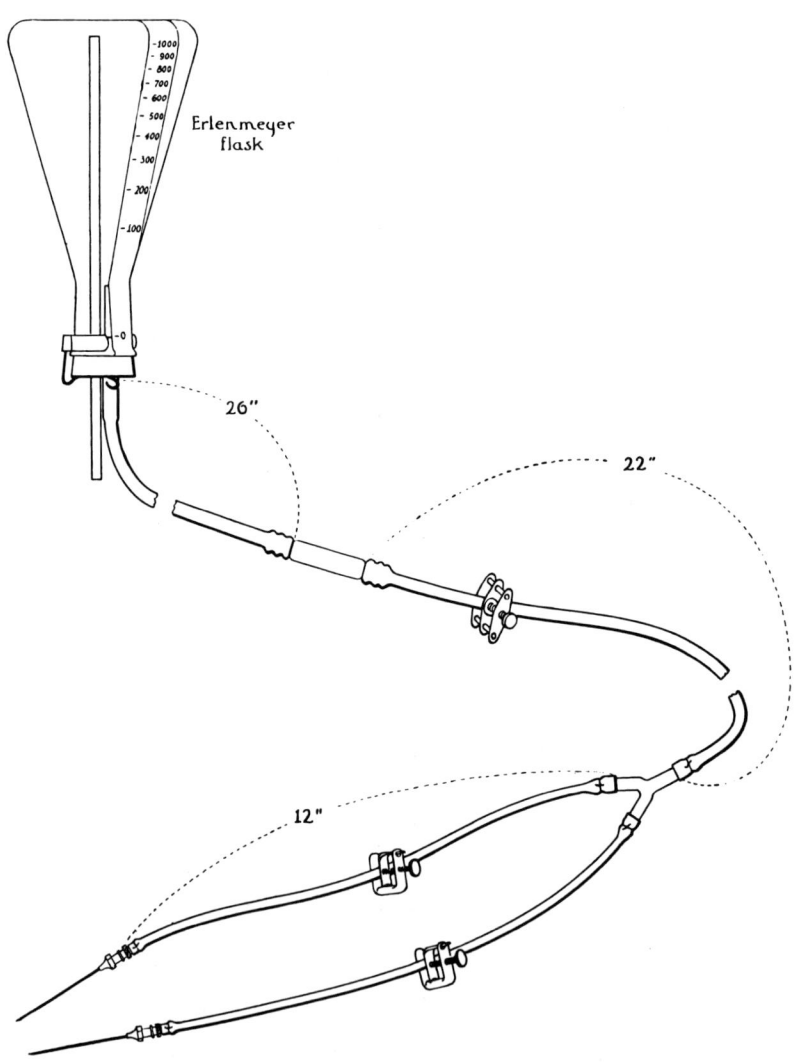

Preparation of equipment
1. Heat solution by setting in basin of water 140° F.
2. Take pins out of tray, but do not uncover.
3. Carry all equipment to bedside.

Preparation of patient
1. Screen completely and explain what treatment is to be. Reassure patient if apprehensive of danger and pain.
2. If thighs are to be used for injection, fold upper covers from just below area to foot of bed. Cover chest and abdomen with bath blanket and another heavy blanket if weather warrants. Place bath towel over pubic region and between legs.
3. If area below breasts is to be used, fold bedding down to below breasts, pin gown up, and cover chest with folded bath blanket.
4. A rubber-covered pillow placed under the knees helps to alleviate discomfort if injection is given in thighs.

Procedure
1. The areas for injection are prepared by the doctor, using sterile applicators and iodine 3.5 per cent and alcohol 70 per cent. One sterile towel is placed over edge of lower bedclothes.
2. The nurse opens tray and places on it the syringe and needles.
3. Pour into medicine glass the amount of novocaine ordered. The doctor injects a small amount subcutaneously with the small hypodermic, and the rest is poured into the flask.
4. Place ring clamp around flask.
5. Remove cover from flask of solution and place in it the rubber stopper, being careful not to contaminate inside of stopper.
6. The metal clamp is screwed in place so as to prevent stopper from falling out.
7. Close screw clamps on tubing and invert flask.
8. After air is expelled from tubes, elevate flask on standard by means of ring clamp.
9. The doctor puts each needle through a gauze square; the nurse holds one while he injects the other.
10. A 6-inch strip of adhesive is wound around hilt of needle and fastened to skin on each side. This holds the needles in place and also the gauze square.
11. The flow should be slow enough not to cause engorgement.
12. Place hot-water bottle around tube and cover with bath towel.
13. Be sure that patient is well covered and unit is neat.

After-care of patient
1. Watch for edema; if it occurs, make flow slower or shut it off for a time.
2. Watch patient's color and pulse closely.

3. To add solution to flask:
   a. Heat solution as previously.
   b. Remove cotton ball from flask and add desired amount of fluid, being sure to replace the stopper. Do not wait until flask is empty before replenishing with fluid, for air would get into the tubing.
4. Refill hot-water bottle every 30 minutes.
5. To discontinue the treatment:
   a. Screen patient.
   b. Shut off flow.
   c. Loosen adhesive tape and remove needles.
   d. Seal punctures with a drop of collodion on a small fluff of cotton.
   e. Place flask and tubing on tray.
   f. Remove blankets and replace covers neatly.
   g. Remove screen and extra equipment and leave unit neat and in order.

After-care of equipment
1. Remove trays from bedside table as soon as treatment has been started.
2. When treatment is finished, clean all articles and replace on tray from Sterile Supply Room.
3. Return it to Sterile Supply Room.
4. Station equipment is cleaned and put away in good condition.

Record
1. When tray is ready write in red ink beside the order in doctor's order book, "Tray set up," with initials.
2. When treatment is finished, check order in margin with red ink, indicating the time.
3. In treatment and medication column: time, amount, kind of solution, novocaine added, treatment, by whom started. Time, amount, kind of solution added. Time, total amount, kind of solution taken when discontinued.
4. In nurse's remarks column: any reaction of patient, discomfort, etc.
5. On graphic sheet: total amount taken, in space opposite "subcutaneous."

References
Harmer, *Principles and Practice of Nursing*, pp. 632–34.
Kelley, *Textbook of Nursing Technique*, pp. 130–32.

Intravenous Infusion

Purpose
1. To restore volume to blood stream following hemorrhage.

2. To stimulate the circulation in shock and collapse.
3. To restore to tissues fluid lost through operation, anhydrating diseases, etc.
4. To dilute poisons, flush kidneys, and carry away toxins in toxemia.
5. To give nutriment in form of glucose; also given in insulin reaction.
6. To obtain more immediate effect than could be obtained by hypodermoclysis.

Solutions used
1. Glucose solution 5–10 per cent.
2. Normal saline.
3. Locke's solution (see hypodermoclysis).
4. Ringer's solution; contains sodium chloride, potassium chloride, and calcium chloride.
5. Dawson's solution; contains sodium chloride and sodium bicarbonate.

Temperature of solution
1. 110° F. when given. (Test over doctor's hand.)

Amount used
1. 50–1000 cc.

METHOD No. 1

Necessary articles
Autoclaved tray from Sterile Supply Room with:
 500 cc. enamel graduate.
 Kelly flask with tubing and clamp.
 Luer-Kaufman syringe, 2 cc.
 Forceps.
 Kidney basin.
 2 sterile towels or puncture sheet for draping.
Skin preparation tray with:
 Kidney basin.
 Container of sterile toothpick applicators.
 Forceps jar with lifting forceps in antiseptic solution.
 Rubber protector with hand towel.
 Wide-mouthed bottle with alcohol 70 per cent.
 Wide-mouthed bottle with iodine 3.5 per cent.
 Tourniquet.
Solution to be given.
Standard.
Intravenous needles, 19x1½ inches, in tubes (autoclaved).
Arm board.

Preparation of equipment
1. Heat solution by placing in basin of warm water (120° F.).
   Place on skin preparation tray.
2. Remove pins from wrapper, but do not uncover tray.
3. Carry all articles to bedside.

Preparation of patient
1. If patient is conscious, make sure he understands nature of
   treatment.
2. See that lighting is adequate; provide extension light if necessary.
3. Place arm board under arm; if patient is unconscious, irrational, or uncooperative, tie wrist down with wide bandage.
4. Fold up sleeve of gown as near shoulder as possible.
5. Place rubber protector under elbow and tourniquet above
   elbow.

Procedure
1. The doctor disinfects the area with iodine and alcohol and
   places the sterile drapes.
2. With tubing clamped, the doctor holds the Kelly flask, and the
   nurse pours in solution.
3. The doctor then connects the syringe to the tubing, the clamp
   is opened, and air is expelled from the tubing, the nurse holding the Kelly flask.
4. It is then hung on the standard from 2 to 2½ feet above the
   patient.
5. Under sterile drape the nurse will apply the tourniquet until
   the doctor indicates that the needle is in the vein, when the
   tourniquet is carefully released and the desired fluid is given.
6. The nurse is not held responsible for the administration of
   any intravenous infusion.
7. Watch the patient for chills, ringing in ears, dizziness, marked
   increase in pulse or respiration.

METHOD No. 2

Necessary articles:
Autoclaved tray from Sterile Supply Room with:
   Rubber tubing with connecting rods and clamp.
   Glass nipple on end to be inserted into bottle containing solu-
   tion.
   Kidney basin.
   Luer-Kaufman syringe, 2 cc.
Bottle of warmed solution with handle. This bottle has in it a
   2-holed rubber stopper. In one hole is a glass tube, which ex-
   tends to ½ inch from bottom of bottle.

Skin preparation tray with articles as listed under method no. 1. Standard.

Preparation of equipment
1. Heat solution by placing in basin of warm water (120° F.). Place on skin preparation tray.
2. Remove pins from wrapper, but do not uncover tray.
3. Carry all articles to bedside.

Preparation of patient
1. If patient is conscious, make sure he understands nature of the treatment.
2. See that lighting is adequate; provide extension light if necessary.
3. Place arm board under arm; if patient is unconscious, irrational, or uncooperative, tie wrist down with wide bandage.
4. Fold up sleeve of gown as near shoulder as possible.
5. Place rubber protector under elbow, and tourniquet above elbow.

Procedure
1. The doctor disinfects area with iodine and alcohol and places sterile drapes.
2. The nurse will remove the metal cap of the solution jar and hold the jar while the doctor removes the washers and inserts the glass nipple.
3. The air is removed from the tubing.
4. The nurse attaches the handle and hangs up the bottle.
5. The doctor then connects the syringe to the tubing, the clamp is opened, and air is expelled from the tubing, the nurse holding the flask.
6. It is then hung on the standard from 2 to 2½ feet above the patient.
7. Under the sterile drape the nurse will apply the tourniquet until the doctor indicates that the needle is in the vein, when the tourniquet is carefully released and the desired fluid is given.
8. The nurse is not held responsible for the administration of any intravenous infusion.
9. Watch the patient for chills, ringing in ears, dizziness, marked increase in pulse or respiration.

After-care of patient
1. Check to see that there is no bleeding from the puncture wound.
2. See that there are no blood stains on patient or on his bedding.
3. Replace gown.

4. Remove screen and other articles and leave unit in order.
5. Keep patient warm and protected from drafts.

After-care of equipment
1. Rinse needles and syringe free from blood before it coagulates.
2. Be sure to remove all glucose (if given) from tubing and rest of apparatus.
3. Return equipment to Sterile Supply Room, clean and in good condition.
4. Give proper care to station equipment and put away in good condition.

Record
1. Treatment column: hour, treatment, amount and kind of solution, by whom, initials of nurse.
2. In nurse's remarks column: reaction of patient to treatment.
3. On graphic sheet: check opposite space for intravenous fluids.

References
Harmer, *Principles and Practice of Nursing*, pp. 626–32.
Kelley, *Textbook of Nursing Technique*, pp. 132–37.

Venisection Tray

Purpose
1. Used with venipuncture, intravenous infusion, and transfusions when the vein is too small or too deeply imbedded in surrounding tissue to be accessible through the skin.

Solution
1. Novocaine 10 per cent.

Necessary articles
Tray.
Sterile articles:
  4 medicine glasses.
  8 cotton balls.
  3 sterile towels.
  2 gauze squares.
  Sterile dermal suture.
  2 curved cutting-edge needles.
  500 cc. graduate.
  2 cc. syringe.
  Hypodermic needles.
  Suture scissors.
  Needle holder.
  2 Kelly forceps.
  2 small cat's-paw retractors.
  Probe.
  Scalpel.

Unsterile articles:
Package sterile gloves.
Adhesive tape ½ inch wide.
Tourniquet.
Rubber protector with hand towel.
Flask of sterile novocaine 1 per cent.

Preparation of equipment
1. Sterilize sharp instruments by placing in disinfecting solution for 20 minutes. Rinse well with sterile water and place on sterile tray.
2. Boil other articles for sterile tray 20 minutes.
3. Collect and arrange all other articles.
4. If treatment is to be given in dressing room, place articles and trays conveniently on table. If done at the bedside, carry equipment to bedside.

Preparation of patient
1. Tell patient what the treatment is to be.
2. Screen completely, if in a ward; if in a room, place screen before door.
3. Expose arm by folding sleeve of gown away from field of treatment close to patient's body.
4. Place covered rubber protector under arm.
5. Place tourniquet under arm about 3 inches above the elbow.
6. Sterilize the skin at the point of insertion of the needle (an area about 4 inches in radius) by cleansing with applicator dipped in iodine and then with alcohol. (The doctor usually does this.)
7. Just before the doctor is ready to start the treatment, open up syringe and needle.
8. Fasten tourniquet as tightly as is necessary to make vein stand out prominently, and in such a manner that the ends of tourniquet are pointed toward patient's shoulder.

Procedure
1. The doctor disinfects the skin area and makes a small incision over the vein through which he makes the puncture with the needle into the vein.
2. The nurse stays with the doctor to see that all his wants are supplied.

After-care of patient
1. Small, dry, sterile dressing applied after treatment is completed.
2. Check to see that there is no bleeding from puncture wound.
3. See that there are no blood stains on patient or on his bedding.

4. Replace gown.
5. Remove screen and other articles and leave unit in order.
6. Keep patient warm and protected from drafts.

After-care of equipment
1. Wash blood from instruments before it coagulates.
2. Separate sharp instruments from other instruments.
3. Boil 3 minutes and put away in proper condition, returning any borrowed articles.

Record
1. In treatment and medication column: time, treatment, doctor.
2. In nurse's remarks column: unusual symptoms and reaction of patient.

References
Harmer, *Principles and Practice of Nursing*, pp. 422–23.
Kelley, *Textbook of Nursing Technique*, pp. 186–87.

Thoracentesis

Purpose
1. To withdraw fluid from the chest for diagnostic or therapeutic purposes.

Necessary articles
Autoclaved tray from Sterile Supply Room, containing:
   Aspirating tube.
   Stopcock and cork with rubber tubes with adaptors attached.
   2 medicine glasses.
   Forceps.
   Large 4-liter bottle.
Flask of novocaine 1 per cent.
Flask of normal saline.
Air pump from Sterile Supply Room.
Skin preparation tray with:
   Container with sterile cotton applicators.
   Container with sterile cotton balls.
   Wide-mouthed bottle with alcohol 3.5 per cent.
   Wide-mouthed bottle with iodine 70 per cent.
   Small rubber sheet and drawsheet.
   Collodion.
   2 sterile test tubes in container.
   Alcohol lamp and matches.
Adhesive.
2 sterile towels.
Sterile gloves.
2 sterile aspirating needles in tubes.

2 sterile hypodermic needles in tubes.

Sterile 2 cc. syringe.

Sterile 20 cc. syringe.

Preparation of equipment

1. Remove pins from wrapper around tray, but leave covered except when removing articles.
2. Remove syringes from wrappers, needles from tubes, and place on sterile tray.
3. Arrange all articles conveniently on table in dressing room, or carry to bedside.

Preparation of patient

1. Procedure may be done either at bedside or in dressing room.
2. Explain purpose and nature of treatment to patient; if in ward, screen completely.
3. Have patient sit on side of bed or table. Place chair in front of him on which he may rest his feet.
4. Place bath blanket folded in triangle around shoulders, pin at back.
5. Place second folded bath blanket over lap and around legs.
6. Remove sleeve of gown on affected side.
7. Bring gown around to opposite side and pin. This makes a holder for the rubber sheet and sterile towel.
8. Place patient's hand on affected side on opposite shoulder.
9. Cover shoulders with small square sheet.
10. Place small rubber sheet in holder made by pinning gown.
11. At and about the point of insertion of needle (designated by the physician) paint the skin with iodine 3.5 per cent. Allow iodine to dry. Then remove iodine with alcohol 70 per cent.

Procedure

1. The doctor prepares the skin area around site of puncture and applies sterile drape.
2. For diagnostic purpose or when only a small amount of fluid is to be withdrawn:
   a. Pour about 4 mils (cc.) of novocaine into sterile medicine glass. The physician will draw the solution into the hypodermic syringe and anesthetize the area about the point of insertion of thoracentesis needle. He then attaches the thoracentesis needle to the syringe, inserts into the pleural cavity, and withdraws fluid.
   b. Light the alcohol lamp ready to flame the rim of one of the sterile tubes when ready to receive the fluid. A second tube may or may not be used.
   c. As the physician withdraws the needle, have a swab and

collodion ready with which to seal the wound. A dressing may be used instead.

3. For therapeutic purpose:

   a. The nurse exhausts the air in the graduated bottle by use of air pump. (Note arrow on nozzle of pump. The arrow on tip attached to bottle must point toward pump.) Pour normal saline into medicine glass, and test bottle for vacuum by placing end of tube in solution and opening valve. The physician anesthetizes area about point of insertion of needle with novocaine.

   b. Bring bottle close to patient. The physician fastens the needle firmly to the sterile rubber tube, then inserts the needle into the pleural cavity.

   c. When directed by the physician, the nurse opens the valve of the tube leading from the patient, and the fluid will flow slowly into the bottle.

   d. Close the wound in the same manner as directed in the preceding method.

After-care of patient

1. Watch patient for signs of collapse, especially when large amounts of fluid are withdrawn.
2. The patient should lie quietly in bed for a number of hours after the treatment.
3. Give fluids by mouth unless contra-indicated.
4. Keep patient warm.

After-care of equipment

1. Be careful that nothing comes in contact with the fluid removed from the thorax, as it often contains organisms of an infectious nature. The nurse must bear in mind that her hands are considered contaminated until she has finished cleaning the equipment and has scrubbed her hands well.
2. The equipment is carefully and thoroughly washed with soap and water, rinsed, and boiled 3 minutes.
3. The equipment is put away clean and in good condition.
4. Equipment from Sterile Supply Room is returned clean and in good order.
5. The specimens must be taken to the laboratory as soon as possible after the treatment.

Record

1. In treatment column: hour, treatment, amount, and character of fluid removed and by whom. Record specimen to laboratory, if sent. Nurse's initials.
2. In nurse's remarks column: reaction of patient to treatment.

References
Harmer, *Principles and Practice of Nursing*, pp. 427–30.
Kelley, *Textbook of Nursing Technique*, pp. 179–81.

Abdominal Paracentesis

Purpose
1. To withdraw fluid from the abdominal cavity for diagnostic or therapeutic purposes.

Necessary articles
To be sterilized and placed on sterile tray:
  8 gauze squares 3x3 inches.
  Sterile towel or spinal drape.
  Sterile abdominal pad.
  Small scalpel.
  Suture scissors.
  Medium-sized trocar and cannula with 8-inch tubing.
  2 medicine glasses.
  2 cc. syringe.
  2 hypodermic needles.
  3-foot rubber tubing with glass connecting tube.
  1 rat-tooth forceps or hemostat.
  Needle holder.
  Preparation forceps.
  2 cutting-edge curved needles.
  Dermal suture.
  500 cc. graduate.
  Kidney basin.
Skin preparation tray with:
  Container of sterile cotton applicators.
  Wide-mouthed bottle of alcohol 70 per cent.
  Wide-mouthed bottle of iodine 3.5 per cent.
  Small rubber sheet with cover.
  Collodion.
  Adhesive ½–1 inch wide.
Glass or other container to hold upright 2 test tubes:
  5 cc. sodium citrate, 2 per cent.
  Empty sterile tube.
Package of sterile gloves.
Flask of novocaine 1 or 2 per cent.
Large pail to collect fluid when large amount is withdrawn.

Preparation of equipment
1. Sterilize sharp instruments by placing in disinfecting solution for 20 minutes. Rinse well with sterile water and place on sterile tray.

2. Boil other articles for sterile tray 20 minutes.
3. Collect and arrange all other articles.
4. If treatment is to be given in dressing room, place articles and trays conveniently on table. If done at bedside carry equipment to bedside.

Preparation of patient

1. Explain nature and purpose of treatment to patient. Screen completely, if in a ward.
2. Have patient empty bladder. A distended bladder might easily be punctured.
3. Shave, if necessary, an area on lower abdomen (4–6 inches square), at and about insertion of the trocar.
4. Have patient sit on a straight-backed chair, if possible. If not, he may sit on side of bed with legs hanging well over the edge, feet resting on a footrest or rungs of a chair, or he may sit up against pillows at head of bed with legs extended straight forward. Bring gown well up under arms and fasten at back.
5. Place small rubber sheet over lap, well against lower abdomen below prepared skin surface.
6. Place a triangularly folded bath blanket around shoulders and pin in front, and a folded blanket over lap and around legs.

Procedure

1. The physician prepares the skin area around site of puncture and applies sterile drapes.
2. The physician anesthetizes the area about the point of insertion of the trocar, then makes a small incision with the scalpel and inserts trocar and cannula. The nurse has ready the flat basin to collect the fluid. A small amount of fluid is allowed to flow into the basin.
3. The nurse removes the plug from a sterile test tube, flames the rim, and holds it ready to receive the fluid. 1 or 2 tubes, as requested, may be used. The remainder of the fluid, or as much as the physician wishes to withdraw, is collected in the basin or pan.
4. As the fluid is being withdrawn, the nurse must observe patient closely for symptoms of collapse.
5. As the physician withdraws trocar and cannula, the nurse has ready a cotton ball for cleansing the wound.
6. If necessary, a few stitches may be taken in the wound.
7. Apply sterile dressings and abdominal pad over wound.
8. Have patient lie down, and put on an abdominal binder snugly.
9. Remove drapes and see that patient is placed in bed in a comfortable position.

After-care of patient
1. Have patient lie in bed quietly for at least 6 hours, or as long as there is any pain or drainage.
2. Keep abdominal binder on, quite tightly, for 1 or 2 days.
3. Watch for chills, headache, abdominal pain, dizziness, respiratory or cardiac difficulty.

After-care of equipment
1. Measure fluid and discard it.
2. The equipment is carefully and thoroughly washed with soap and water, rinsed, and boiled 3 minutes.
3. The equipment is put away clean and in good condition.
4. The specimens must be taken to the laboratory as soon as possible after the treatment.

Record
1. In treatment column: hour, treatment, amount and character of fluid removed, by whom. Record specimen to laboratory, if sent. Nurse's initials.
2. In nurse's remarks column: reaction of patient to treatment.
3. Record with output: date and amount.

References
Harmer, *Principles and Practice of Nursing*, pp. 432–34.
Kelley, *Textbook of Nursing Technique*, pp. 181–83.

Spinal Puncture

Purpose
1. To withdraw fluid for diagnostic or therapeutic purposes.
2. To administer medications, as sera.

Solution
Novocaine 1 per cent.

Necessary articles
On sterile half of tray:
2 spinal puncture needles, 1 large, 1 small.
2 hypodermic needles.
1 medicine glass.
1 spinal drape or 2 sterile towels.
Spinal monometer.
Forceps.
2 cc. syringe.
Kidney basin.
Note. — If treatment is being given for the purpose of injecting serum, add to the tray:
20 cc. syringe.
500 cc. graduate.

On unsterile half of tray:

3 sterile spinal puncture tubes labeled 1, 2, and 3, with adhesive tape, held upright in a paper box.

Small rubber square, covered with towel.

Package of sterile towels.

Laboratory request sheets.

Collodion.

Preparation of equipment

1. All equipment that is to be sterile is wrapped and boiled 20 minutes.
2. The technique of setting up the tray is that used in setting up any tray when half is sterile.
3. If treatment is to be given in dressing room, arrange trays conveniently on table; if in a ward, carry articles to bedside.
4. Arrange chair or stool for doctor to use.

Preparation of patient

1. Explain nature of treatment to patient and the necessity and value of his cooperation.
2. Screen completely, if in a ward; if in a room, place screen before door.
3. Remove pillows from head. Have patient lie on side and near edge of bed. Flex the body, bringing chin as close to knees as possible. (This position arches the body, brings out the spinal processes, and opens the interspaces between the processes.)
4. Bring gown around to front and pin.
5. Place folded bath blanket around shoulders and another blanket, kind depending on temperature of the room, around hips and legs.

Procedure

1. Protect bed with small rubber sheet.
2. Expose lower half of back and doctor will disinfect skin area with iodine and alcohol.
3. Sterile drapes are placed around the field. It is sometimes necessary to pin these in place. When the treatment is given at bedside, remove all the pillows and have patient lie on side near edge of bed. Replace covers with a bath blanket.
4. Pour the novocaine just before doctor is ready to use it, telling him what you are pouring and the percentage.
5. The doctor injects the local anesthetic.
6. The doctor inserts the needle. The nurse, just before the stilette is removed from the needle, selects sterile tube no. 1, removes the plug by touching only the top, flames the rim of the tube, and holds ready to collect fluid. Usually about 2

fluid drams is collected. Tubes 2 and 3 are used in the same way if 3 tubes are used.

7. As the doctor withdraws the needle, the nurse has the collodion and swab ready. The wound is sealed with the collodion. No dressing is used.

8. Watch patient during procedure and notify the doctor at once if patient complains of faintness, headache, nausea, or ringing in ears, or if you notice respiratory embarrassment or any change in pulse beat.

After-care of patient

1. Put patient back to bed, causing as little exertion as possible.
2. Instruct patient to lie on his back without a pillow for 8 hours.
3. The patient may have a pillow after 8 hours, but should stay in bed for 24 hours.
4. The diet may be the usual diet, but in feeding patient while he is on his back and without a pillow, give any assistance necessary.

After-care of equipment

1. The specimen tubes are properly labeled and taken to laboratory immediately after the treatment.
2. Equipment is washed and boiled for 3 minutes and put away as previously instructed.

Record

1. Treatment column: hour, treatment, amount of fluid taken, surgeon, specimen to laboratory, initials of nurse.
2. Nurse's remarks column: unusual symptoms and reaction of patient.

References

Harmer, *Principles and Practice of Nursing*, pp. 435–41.
Kelley, *Textbook of Nursing Technique*, pp. 176–79.

V. STERILE FOMENTATIONS

Purpose
1. To apply heat and moisture to a part.
2. To apply heat in accordance with aseptic technic.
3. To apply moist dressings so as to cause as little pain and discomfort as possible.

General instructions
1. The dry sterile flannel is the dividing line between the sterile and unsterile material used.
2. Hot-water bottles must be changed at least every 2 hours in order to insure a sufficient degree of heat to make the treatment efficacious.
3. Dressings must be kept well moistened.
4. Use large enough rubber protector to insure that bed is protected and to prevent circulation of air around wet compresses.

Types
1. Abdominal.
2. Extremities or any other part of body.

Necessary articles
Dressing cart or tray with:
  Container with sterile flannels.
  Container with sterile fluffs.
  Covered pitcher.
  Rubber protector or oiled muslin (used for hot packs only).
  Hot-water bags.
  Cover for pack — binder, muslin, etc.
  Safety pins.
  Sterile lifter in solution.
  Sterile forceps or hemostats in container.
  Kidney basin for used forceps.
  Newspaper for waste.

Preparation of equipment
1. Prepare sterile solution at 115° F.
2. Fill hot-water bottles one-third full at 130° F.; do not cover.
3. Take cart or tray to bedside.

To Apply to Abdomen

Preparation of patient
1. Wash your hands.
2. Tell patient what the treatment is to be.
3. Screen completely in the routine way.

4. Fold top bedding down to pubes.
5. Fold gown back over chest; if ward is cold, the bath blanket should be used over the chest.
6. Open binder if patient has one.
7. Place newspaper, unfolded, on bed. Loosen adhesive and remove top pad if there is an incision.

Procedure
1. With sterile lifter remove hemostat from container.
2. Remove dressings from incision.
3. With sterile lifter in one hand and hemostat in other, remove dressing from can and apply unfolded over incision.
4. Moisten with solution from pitcher.
5. Remove sterile flannel from container, place over dressings, and moisten.
6. Remove second sterile flannel, place over moistened flannel. Do not moisten this flannel; the outer layer should remain dry.
7. Cover with rubber protector or oiled muslin.
8. Place hot-water bottle. Be sure that bottle does not touch the skin.
9. Bring up binder and pin.
10. Fold gown down.
11. Pull top bedding up.
12. Remove cart.
13. After two hours wash hands well, open fomentation down to sterile moist flannel, and moisten with solution at 115° F.
14. Refill hot-water bottle.

To Apply to Extremity

Preparation of patient
1. Loosen bedding if necessary and place extremity outside of bedclothes.
2. If dressings are present, remove in same manner as abdominal ones.

Procedure
1. Place binder on bed.
2. Place rubber protector on binder.
3. With sterile lifter remove sterile flannel and place over rubber.
4. Remove second flannel and place over first.
5. Gently raise extremity and place material under it.
6. In the same way as for the abdomen, remove dressings from container and place over wound so as to make a copious dressing.

7. If wound is on under side of extremity, dressings are placed on the flannel before it is put under extremity.
8. Moisten dressings with solution.
9. Bring up first flannel with hemostat and moisten.
10. Bring up second flannel, the inside of which is sterile.
11. Bring up rubber protector.
12. Place hot-water bottles, bring up binder and pin.

After-care of patient when fomentations are discontinued
1. Bring dressing cart to bedside.
2. Using aseptic technique, remove wet flannel and dressings.
3. Apply dry fluffs and fasten binder.

After-care of equipment
1. Flannels are changed every day and sent to the laundry.
2. Cart should be replenished with materials after each use.
3. Gauze, on removal, is put in pail for waste gauze.

Record
1. In treatment and medication column: time, type, how long continued, reaction, results, and initials.
2. In nurse's remarks column: general effect, comfort or discomfort.

References
Harmer, *Principles and Practice of Nursing*, pp. 244–50.

VI. VAGINAL IRRIGATION (DOUCHE)

Purpose
1. To cleanse the vaginal tract of
   a. irritating or profuse discharge.
   b. source of odor.
2. To relieve inflammation.
3. To check hemorrhage (very rarely).

General instructions
1. When method no. 1 is used for giving a hot solution, avoid burning patient by coating perineum and region around anus with vaseline.
2. The length of time required for giving the solution is important; when used to relieve inflammation, the rate of flow should be regulated to a maximum of 15 minutes to 2000 cc.
3. During catamenia, douches are discontinued unless ordered by the doctor.
4. Use extreme care if there are stitches in the perineum.
5. Be sure that douche nozzle is not cracked or broken.
6. The patient is not allowed to insert the douche point or take her own douche.

Solutions usually ordered
1. Tap water; allow water to flow from tap for 1 minute, so as to insure cleanliness.
2. Normal saline.
3. Lysol or cresolis compositus solution 0.5 per cent.
4. Sodium bicarbonate 2 per cent.
5. Potassium permanganate 1/10–1 per cent.
6. Bichloride of mercury 1/3000–1/10,000.
7. Normal saline with sodium bicarbonate 2 per cent.
8. A. B. C. powder (alum, boric, calomel) 1 teaspoonful to 1 quart of water.

Temperature of solution
1. For cleansing and deodorizing, 105° F.
2. For inflammation, 115° F.
3. For hemorrhage, 130°–140° F.

Amount of solution
1. 1 quart–1 gallon.

Necessary articles
Standard.
Douche can with tubing.
Sterile dressing towel.

2 sterile cotton balls.

Douche pan.

Sterile perineal pad.

Kidney basin.

Bath thermometer.

Douche point or mon docteur.

Large sheet or bath blanket.

Rubber protector.

2 bedpan covers.

1000 cc. sterile graduate.

Sterile forceps.

Hemostat.

Kidney basin.

Tray.

METHOD No. 1, USING GLASS DOUCHE POINT

Preparation of equipment

1. Place douche can, tubing, kidney basin, hemostat, douche point, and graduate in sterilizer; boil 10 minutes.
2. Remove articles from sterilizer and arrange on tray.
3. Place douche point, hemostat, and cotton balls in kidney basin, cover with sterile towel, and place on tray.
4. Prepare solution of correct amount, strength, and temperature in graduate, pour into can.
5. Place covered rubber protector, perineal pad, and sheet for draping (unless kept at bedside) on tray.
6. Cover tray and carry to bedside. Place on bedside table.
7. Carry in standard and warmed douche pan. Place douche pan on chair.

Preparation of patient

1. Tell patient what the treatment is to be.
2. Screen patient completely, if in a ward; if in a room, place screen before door.
3. Have patient void before giving douche.
4. Fanfold covers to foot of bed and replace with bath blanket.
5. Drape well with bath blanket and if ward is cold, as at night, place a woolen blanket over chest and abdomen.
6. Remove pillows from under head. If patient is too uncomfortable, one pillow may be left.
7. Uncover tray. Hang cover over head of bed.
8. Place rubber protector, covered with bedpan cover, under hips.
9. Uncover douche pan, hang cover over foot of bed, and place pan under hips.

Procedure

1. Hang can on standard about 2 feet above patient. If can block is used, move table about to middle of bed, place can block on tray and irrigating can on block.
2. Put finger cots on thumb and forefinger of left hand.
3. Separate labia and cleanse external genitalia with flow of solution from the tubing.

4. Place kidney basin, containing douche point, on bed between patient's feet.
5. Examine douche point and connect to rubber tubing.
6. Insert gently downward and backward into vagina.
7. Regulate flow so that there will be little pressure from the solution.
8. Gently rotate and move douche point forward and backward along vaginal tract so that all parts will be cleaned.
9. Continue treatment until prescribed amount of solution has been used.
10. Disconnect point, examine to see that it is still intact, place in kidney basin.
11. Dry labia with cotton balls held in hemostat.
12. Place kidney basin on tray.
13. Remove douche pan.
14. Using cover under patient, dry buttocks well.
15. Place perineal pad.
16. Remove protector and drape and replace bed covers.
17. Remove screen, cover tray, and carry out equipment.

METHOD NO. 2, USING "MON DOCTEUR" DOUCHE POINT

Preparation of equipment
1. Boil equipment as in method no. 1.
2. Place irrigator in kidney basin and pour over it cold sterile water to insure that it will be cool before it is used.
3. Prepare rest of equipment as in method no. 1.

Preparation of patient: same as in method no. 1.

Procedure
1. Hang can on standard about 2 feet above patient. If can block is used, move table about to middle of bed, place can block on tray and irrigating can on block.
2. Put finger cots on thumb and forefinger of left hand.
3. Separate labia and cleanse external genitalia with flow of solution from tubing.
4. Place kidney basin, containing douche point, on bed between patient's feet.
5. Examine douche point to see that rubber point is pushed well up into porcelain portion.
6. Clamp outflow tube shut with hemostat.
7. Attach rubber tubing from can to inflow.
8. Separate labia and insert point as far as possible. The flat side of the porcelain portion should be flush with the outer vaginal orifice. The insertion and use of this irrigator should not cause discomfort.

9. Open stopcock and allow solution to flow into vagina.
10. Let outflow tube remain clamped off for approximately 10 seconds, or until solution begins to return around porcelain.
11. Open clamp on outflow and allow to drain into douche pan.
12. Allow irrigation to continue until all of solution is used.
13. Finish procedure as in steps 10–16 in method no. 1.

After-care of patient
1. Have patient remain quiet and in bed for at least an hour following treatment.

After-care of equipment
1. Wash and dry can and rubber tubing, replace on shelf.
2. Boil douche point and replace.
3. Discard cotton balls and place soiled linen in hamper.

Record
1. In treatment and medication column: time, treatment, kind and amount of solution used, returns (as containing mucus, pus, etc.).
2. In nurse's remarks column: comfort or discomfort caused by treatment.
3. Nurse's initials follow all recording.

References
Harmer, *Principles and Practice of Nursing*, pp. 348–53.
Kelley, *Textbook of Nursing Technique*, pp. 103–10.

VII. CATHETERIZATION AND RELATED PROCEDURES

Purpose
  Catheterization: To remove urine from the bladder.
  Instillation: To place healing and antiseptic solutions in bladder.
  Irrigation: To wash out bladder with antiseptic solution.

General instructions
  1. Never catheterize without an order.
  2. Use every known means to get patient to void first unless special orders are given following some operation or treatment.

Necessary articles
  Sterile catheter carrier containing:
      2 metal catheters no. 14 with 2 inches of rubber tubing attached.
      Large cotton applicator.
      Gauze sponge.
  Bag containing sterile solution basin and 7 large toothpick cotton applicators.
  Large basin (800 cc.) for urine.
  Small kidney basin for waste.
  Box containing several clean, powdered finger cots.
  Rubber protector and bedpan cover.
  Tube of lubricant.

Preparation of equipment
  1. Secure catheter carrier and sterile solution basin from Sterile Supply Room.
  2. Untie bandage from around catheter carrier and place on tray.
  3. Open bag and remove solution basin. Pour approximately 200 cc. of a solution of bichloride of mercury 1/1000 and sodium oleate 0.2 per cent. Place on tray.
  4. Disinfect top of lubricant tube by wiping top with applicator dipped in the bichloride solution and let approximately an inch of lubricant fall on gauze sponge in catheter carrier.
  5. Arrange with other articles on tray.
  6. Cover tray with dressing towel.
  7. Wash hands well and dry, carry tray in, place on bedside chair.

Preparation of patient
  1. Tell patient what the treatment is to be.
  2. Screen completely if in a ward; if in a room, place screen before door.
  3. Fanfold top bedding down and replace with bath blanket.

4. Drape patient as for pelvic examination; if ward is cold, as at night, place a woolen blanket over chest and abdomen.
5. Place tray between feet at foot of bed.
6. Uncover tray and place rubber covered protector well under hips.

Procedure
1. Put finger cots from box on thumb and forefinger of left hand; if labia are swollen or difficult to hold back it may be necescary to protect more than two fingers.
2. Place large basin in position to receive urine.
3. Separate labia with fingers of left hand and with 5 cotton applicators cleanse well around meatus.
4. Open catheter carrier. Pick up catheter near end; be sure that at least 2 inches of tip is well lubricated and uncontaminated for 4 inches.
5. Insert lubricated catheter gently and slowly approximately 2 inches, until urine is obtained.
6. A metal catheter slides easily, so it is usually necessary to hold it in place to prevent its slipping out.
7. When there is no more urine in bladder, remove catheter and place in waste basin.
8. Cleanse meatus with cotton applicator from solution.
9. Dry around meatus and labia with dry cotton applicator from catheter carrier.
10. Remove finger cots.
11. Place basin of urine on tray.
12. Remove covered rubber protector and dry buttocks well with cover; place on tray.
13. Cover tray and remove to chair at foot of bed.
14. Remove drape and bring up covers.
15. Remake covers at foot of bed and leave bed in good order.
16. Remove screen.
17. Carry out tray.

After-care of patient
1. Be sure patient is warm and dry following treatment.
2. Try to induce voluntary micturition before bladder becomes distended again.

After-care of equipment
1. Wash finger cots with soap and water, boil 5 minutes, dry, powder, and replace in box.
2. Wash emesis basins, boil 5 minutes, dry, and replace on tray.
3. Wash catheters well with soap and water, dry, replace in carrier on clean gauze square.

4. Wash solution basin with soap and water, put in bag, tie opening with 1-inch bandage, and send to Sterile Supply Room.
5. Replace 1 large cotton swab in carrier. Put on cover and tie with piece of 1-inch bandage. Send to Sterile Supply Room for autoclaving.
6. Wash rubber protector, dry, cover with clean bedpan cover, fold, and replace on tray.

Note on care of metal catheters. — They can and must be kept scrupulously clean. They should occasionally be cleaned on the inside with a small applicator and should always be dried well when put back into carrier for sterilization.

Record

1. In treatment and medication column: time, treatment, retention, specimen to laboratory.
2. In nurse's remarks column: pain caused by treatment, relief obtained, or any other observation made.
3. Nurse's initials follow all recording.

Related procedures

1. Catheterization for specimen
   a. Place corked bottle on tray.
   b. Proceed according to previous instructions.
   c. Just before putting on finger cots, uncork bottle.
   d. Before inserting catheter, place bottle conveniently near patient.
   e. If sterile specimen is ordered, boil bottle for 5 minutes and stopper with a sterile cotton ball. Place second sterile cotton ball in carrier, which will be used as a stopper after specimen is obtained.
2. Bladder instillation
   a. Obtain from Sterile Supply Room instillation set which contains 2 metal catheters, barrel of aseptic syringe, medicine glass, and gauze sponge.
   b. Include on tray the bottle containing medication ordered.
   c. Proceed as for catheterization.
   d. After urine is withdrawn, remove medicine glass from carrier, place on tray, and pour into it the amount ordered for instillation.
   e. Attach barrel of syringe to rubber on catheter and pour in solution.
   f. Elevate until all of medication has gone into bladder.
   g. Chart as for catheterization, including kind, strength, and amount of medication used.

3. Bladder irrigation
   a. Obtain from Sterile Supply Room the same set as for instillation and bag containing solution basin and 1000 cc. granite graduate.
   b. Set up tray as for instillation. Add a large basin for return flow.
   c. Pour amount of solution to be used for irrigation into sterile graduate and cover with doubled sterile towel.
   d. Proceed as for catheterization.
   e. After urine has drained from bladder, attach barrel of syringe, pour solution into it, elevate, and continue pouring until 350–400 cc. has been introduced unless patient experiences too much discomfort.
   f. Lower barrel and allow solution to drain out, using care that end of barrel does not touch basin.
   g. Raise barrel and repeat process until amount ordered has been used.
   h. Chart as for catheterization, including amount, kind, and strength of solution used.
4. Catheterization of ante partum patients in active labor or others for whom a metal catheter cannot be used.
   a. Secure same material from Sterile Supply Room as for catheterization, but catheter carrier which is labeled "A. P." This contains same material as others except that it has no catheters in it and contains a hemostat.
   b. Boil 3 firm, rubber catheters, size Fr. 14, for 3 minutes.
   c. Set up tray as for other catheterizations.
   d. Remove catheters from boiler and place in carrier with tips on dressing.
   e. Lubricate catheters as usual and cover.
   f. The technique is the same as for other catheterizations except that hemostat is used to hold catheter while inserting, holding about 2 inches from tip of catheter.
   g. If great difficulty is encountered in inserting catheter, a pair of sterile gloves may be used, but this should be necessary only in a very few cases.

References
Harmer, *Principles and Practice of Nursing*, pp. 652–62.
Kelley, *Textbook of Nursing Technique*, pp. 149–54.

VIII. GENERAL APPLICATIONS OF HEAT AND COLD

The Sponge Bath

Purpose
1. To improve the circulation and respiration.
2. To increase elimination.
3. To relieve restlessness and make the patient more comfortable.
4. To lower the temperature.

General instructions
1. Do not allow patient to be in a draft.
2. Encourage patient to breathe deeply during the treatment.
3. Give plenty of cool water unless contra-indicated.
4. Apply cold to the head.
5. Apply heat to the feet to prevent chilling and to counterbalance temperature between central and peripheral portions of the body.
6. Use friction for the same reason as for the application of heat to the feet.
7. During any of the treatments, watch for evidence of shock:
   a. Weak, irregular pulse.
   b. Pallor about the mouth.
   c. Cyanosis of fingernails.
   d. Slow and shallow respirations.
8. In case of shock, stop treatment, apply external heat, and report condition to head nurse at once.
9. Mop water from bed at intervals during sponge.
10. Sponge is given whenever the temperature is 102.6° F. or whenever ordered.

Necessary articles
Rubber sheet the length of mattress.
Cotton drawsheet.
Hot-water bottle and cover.
Icecap and cover or ice compresses.
Foot tub half full of water at temperature ordered, usually 78°–85° F. (May begin with water at 85° and gradually lower to 75°.)
Bath thermometer.
Bath blanket.
2 bath towels.
Face towel.
Cracked ice.
2 large loose sponges of gauze (1 yard).

191

Preparation of equipment
1. Prepare tub of water at temperature ordered.
2. Carry tub with other articles to bedside.

Preparation of patient
1. Tell patient what the treatment is to be.
2. Screen completely in the routine way.
3. Fanfold top bedding down and replace with bath blanket.
4. Turn patient on side, face away from you.
5. Pass the rubber sheet covered with drawsheet under patient.
6. Place bath towel over pubic area.
7. Remove gown.
8. Place icecap at head and hot-water bottle at feet.

Procedure
1. Sponge face and dry with face towel.
2. Fold back blanket, exposing half of body from neck to foot.
3. Proceed to sponge, using long, even strokes.
4. Begin high on neck (hair line), sponge down over shoulder outer surface of arm.
5. Turn sponge in hand, begin at hair line, and sponge over shoulder and inner arm.
6. Change sponge; beginning at the axilla, sponge down side and over outer surface of thigh to foot.
7. Turn sponge in hand; begin at axilla and sponge down side and over inner surface of thigh to foot.
8. Continue, changing sponge each second stroke, until exposed surface of body has been covered. Continue for 7 or 8 minutes.
9. Then fold bath blanket over sponged surface, exposing other half of body.
10. Proceed in same way for 7 or 8 minutes.
11. Cover patient with bath blanket and turn on side, face away from you.
12. Begin at hair line and sponge length of back to feet. Continue for about 6 minutes.
13. Turn patient on back and leave wrapped in wet blanket and sheet for 10 minutes.

After-care of patient
1. Turn patient on side, face away from you.
2. Roll sheet and rubber sheet close to back.
3. Dry back if necessary.
4. Turn patient on to dry bed and quickly remove rubber and sheet.
5. Complete drying the body if necessary.
6. An alcohol sponge can be given if it adds to patient's comfort.
7. Replace gown.

8. Pull up cover and remove bath blanket.
9. Remove screen and leave unit in order.
10. Remove articles to service room.
11. Take temperature, pulse, and respiration half hour after completion of bath.

After-care of equipment
1. Wash tub with soap and water and boil.
2. Dry and replace on shelf.
3. Wash rubber sheet and dry.
4. Place soiled linen in hamper.

Record
1. In treatment and medication column: time, type of treatment, temperature of application, how long continued, reaction to or effects of treatment, nurse's initials.
2. In nurse's remarks column: acceptance of treatment, general effect.
3. On temperature sheet: indicate with dotted line from temperature taken previous to bath, and dot the drop obtained. Chart treatment below dot, beginning at temperature line.

References
Harmer, *Principles and Practice of Nursing*, pp. 470–71.

The Alcohol Sponge Bath

Purpose
1. To improve the circulation and respiration.
2. To increase elimination.
3. To relieve restlessness and make patient more comfortable.
4. To lower the temperature.

General instructions
1. Given when you wish to disturb patient as little as possible.
2. See "The Sponge Bath," page 191.

Necessary articles
4 bath towels.
Bath blanket.
Icebag and cover.
Hot-water bag and cover.
Gauze sponge.
1 pint alcohol 25 per cent.

Preparation of equipment
1. Pour 1 pint alcohol 25 per cent into hand basin.
2. Carry with other articles to bedside.

Preparation of patient
1. Tell patient what the treatment is to be.

2. Screen completely in the routine way.
3. Fanfold top bedding down and replace with bath blanket.
4. Remove the gown.
5. Place bath towel over pubes.
6. Place second bath towel under one arm and close to and under side.
7. Place third towel under the other side.
8. Place fourth towel under legs and feet, bringing it well up under hips.
9. Place icecap at head and the hot-water bottle at feet.

Procedure
1. Expose half of body from neck to feet and sponge in the same way as in giving the sponge bath, but press the solution from the sponge so that none will drip on the bed.
2. Continue until the entire anterior surface is covered.
3. Turn patient on side.
4. Begin at hair line and sponge length of back to feet.
5. The duration of the bath is 20 minutes.
6. If patient is very weak or movement is difficult, do not turn on side but cool the back by moistening the palms in the solution and slipping them under the back.

After-care of patient
1. Remove the bath towels.
2. Dry the skin if necessary.
3. Replace gown.
4. Pull up covers and remove bath blanket.
5. Remove screen and leave unit in order.
6. Remove articles to service room.
7. Take temperature, pulse, and respiration half hour after completion of bath.

After-care of equipment
1. The alcohol may be used again for the same patient; otherwise it is discarded.
2. Wash and boil basin, dry, and replace on shelf.
3. Place bath towels in hamper.
4. Put gauze sponge in pail for waste gauze.

Record
Same as for sponge bath.

Sedative Pack

Purpose
1. To induce sleep.
2. To prevent exhaustion in the too active or restless patient.
3. To increase elimination through the skin.

Temperatures
48° F., for robust patients who are excited and flushed.
60°–70° F., for patients of average vitality who are restless and sleepless.
92°–97° F., for the frail patient.

General instructions
1. Have the room warm (72° F.) and free from drafts, but supplied with fresh air.
2. See that there are no air pockets in the wet sheet. Have the dry blankets completely wrapped about patient to exclude all air. Air pockets increase the initial chilliness and discomfort.
3. If patient's color or pulse is poor at the end of 10 or 15 minutes, remove from pack, cover with blankets, and give hot drink.
4. Old age and cardiac conditions are definite contra-indications for this treatment.
5. Give patient water to drink as he desires throughout procedure.
6. The light in the room should be subdued.

Necessary articles
Large rubber sheet or mackintosh.
2 large gray blankets.
2 cotton drawsheets.
Tub of water.
Bath thermometer.
Hot-water bottle and cover.
Face towel.
Bath towel.
Feeding cup filled with drinking water.
2 bath blankets.
Icecap and cover.

Preparation of equipment
1. To prepare the blankets:
   a. Place rubber mackintosh on top of bath blanket.
   b. Place first wool blanket crosswise on rubber.
   c. Place second wool blanket lengthwise on first wool blanket.
   d. Fanfold the whole in quarters on both sides to center so that open edge is on outside.
   e. Fold in half with open edges on inside.
   f. Fold second bath blanket the same as bath blanket used in giving a bath.
2. To fold sheets:
   a. Fold one sheet as indicated in step f.
   b. Fold second sheet the same as in steps d and e.

3. Prepare icecap and hot-water bag.
4. Fill tub with water at correct temperature.
5. Immerse cotton sheet in water.
6. Wring sheets thoroughly dry and pour out water.
7. Replace cotton sheets in tub.
8. Place folded blankets, mackintosh, icecap, hot-water bottle, and towels in tub.
9. Carry tub and other articles to bedside.

Preparation of patient
1. Tell patient what the treatment is to be.
2. Screen completely in the routine way.
3. Offer bedpan or allow patient to go to toilet.
4. Place towels, icecap, and hot-water bottle on table.
5. Remove pillows and place on chair.
6. Fanfold top bedding down and replace with bath blanket.
7. Place bath towel over pubic area.
8. Remove patient's gown and place on chair.
9. Turn patient on side with face away from you.
10. Place cotton blanket, rubber mackintosh, and gray blankets under patient.
11. Place hot-water bottle at feet and icecap at head.

Procedure
1. Turn patient on side with face away from you.
2. Place wet sheet folded lengthwise under patient, covering shoulders and arms. Tuck in between arms and limbs so that no body surfaces touch.
3. Replace bath blanket over patient with wet sheet folded crosswise. Tuck in at sides, leave feet out of pack.
4. Fold inside gray blanket down over shoulders.
5. Fold sides over patient, left over right.
6. Fold second gray blanket over patient, left over right, and tuck in at side.
7. Place face towel under chin and over blankets.
8. Bring bed covering over patient.
9. Take temporal pulse every 15 minutes and record.
10. Remain with the patient throughout the pack, if possible.
11. Leave patient in pack as long as he is quiet and comfortable. (The patient is usually comfortable during the neutral stage. This varies from ½ to 3½ hours.)

After-care of patient
1. Fanfold top bedding down.
2. Unfold the 2 woolen blankets from over patient.
3. Replace top wet sheet with bath blanket.

4. Turn patient on side with face away from you.
5. Fold up wet bottom sheet, gray blanket, and rubber mackintosh, remove and place in tub.
6. Leave patient on dry bath blanket.
7. Replace gown.
8. Bring bed covering over patient.
9. Remove icecap and hot-water bottle.
10. Remove screen.
11. Leave patient comfortable and unit in order.
12. Carry tub and other articles to service room.

After-care of equipment
1. Place blankets and sheets with soiled linen.
2. Wash hot-water bottle with soap and water, dry, inflate, and replace on shelf.
3. Clean tub and replace on shelf.
4. Wash rubber mackintosh, dry, roll, and replace in space provided.

Record
1. In treatment column: time given, treatment, length of pack.
2. In nurse's column: effect of treatment.
3. Nurse's initials follow all recording.

References
Mock, Pemberton, and Coulter, *Principles and Practice of Physical Therapy.*
Wright, *Hydrotherapy in Hospitals for Mental Diseases.*

The Sitz Bath

Purpose
1. To relieve tenesmus·in uterine and renal colic.
2. To relax the sphincter of the bladder and overcome retention of urine.
3. To relieve sciatica.
4. To relieve pain, congestion, and inflammation in the organs of the pelvis.
5. To restore the menstrual function.
6. To relieve painful hemorrhoids.

Necessary articles
Sitz tub.
Foot tub.
3 blankets.
Icecap or cold compress.
Thermometer.
3 bath towels.

Water in sitz tub 106°–120° F.
Water in foot tub 110°–120° F.

Preparation of equipment
1. Have bathroom warm.
2. Cover chair with bath blanket and bath towel.
3. Prepare the tubs of water, one at 106° F. and one at 110° F. (see above).
4. Place bath towel over edge of tub.

Preparation of patient
1. Take patient to bathroom unless tub is portable.
2. Remove gown and bathrobe.
3. Drape other bath blanket around shoulders with open side at back.
4. Pin blanket at neck.
5. Place cold applications to head.

Procedure
1. Have patient sit in sitz tub with feet in foot tub.
2. Be sure that patient is immersed from waist to well below thighs.
3. Cover limbs and feet with second blanket, being sure that the tubs are enclosed in the blankets.
4. Duration of bath, 3–10 minutes, or as long as ordered.
5. Increase temperature of water in tubs up to 120° F. or as hot as patient can stand it.
6. Watch pulse and general condition of patient.

After-care of patient
1. When bath is completed, assist patient from tub and dry external genitals and thighs.
2. Put on slippers.
3. Have her sit on chair and put on her bathrobe as you remove the bath blanket.
4. Take patient back to her room and put her to bed.
5. Clean tubs and leave room in perfect order.

Record
1. In treatment and medication column: time, treatment, duration.
2. In nurse's remarks column: reaction, relief obtained, etc.
3. Nurse's initials follow all recording.

References
Kelley, *Textbook of Nursing Technique*, pp. 74–76.
Sanders, *Modern Methods in Nursing*, pp. 97–98.

Colloid Baths

Purpose
1. To relieve skin irritation.

Medications usually ordered
1. Starch: One pound of cornstarch to a bathtub two-thirds full of water. Mix the starch into a smooth paste with cold water. Hot water is then added to this. Boil for 2 minutes and add to bath water.
2. Bran bath: Place 2 pounds of bran in a loose muslin bag, tie, and place in a deep basin. Pour boiling water over it and let it stand 10–15 minutes. Press the moisture from the bag and add all the fluid to the bath solution.
3. Oatmeal and soda: Boil 3 cups of oatmeal in 2 quarts of water until a porridge is formed. Cool. Fill tub half full of water and dissolve in it 1 teacupful of baking soda. Pour the oatmeal porridge into a cheesecloth bag; tie securely and by washing it about in the water dissolve out the mucilaginous material, leaving the residue in the bag. The water should be whitish and opalescent. The bag may be used in washing the scales from the body.
4. Sodium bicarbonate (alkaline bath): Use 8 ounces of bicarbonate of soda to every gallon of water. Dissolve the powder in warm water and add to the bath. Then proceed as above.

Temperature of solution
1. 95°–100° F. Keep constant.

Duration of bath
1. From 10 to 30 minutes.

Procedure
1. Have bathroom temperature not lower than 80° F.
2. Prepare tub with medication ordered.
3. Assist patient to step in and out of tub.
4. Never allow a weak patient to take the bath unassisted. An orderly will assist the male patient.
5. When the patient leaves the tub, dry the skin gently by patting and apply emollient ordered.
6. Clean the bathtub thoroughly.

Record
1. In medication and treatment column: time, type of bath, duration, purpose.
2. In nurse's remarks column: effect on patient if observable.
3. Nurse's initials follow all recording.

References

Harmer, *Principles and Practice of Nursing*, pp. 473–74.
Kelley, *Textbook of Nursing Technique*, pp. 163–64.

Local Hot Water Bath

Purpose
1. To aid in the treatment of infected wounds.

General instructions
1. Avoid burning patient.
2. Maintain a constant temperature, as ordered by physician.
3. Place patient in comfortable position.
4. Use sterile solution when there is an open wound.

Necessary articles
Arm bathtub.
Dressing towel.
Small rubber sheet ⎫
Small blanket ⎭ When a foot tub is used.
Required solution at a temperature 105°–115° F. unless otherwise ordered by physician.

Preparation of equipment
1. Fill tub three-quarters full of solution ordered at the correct temperature. Use thermometer.
2. Arrange articles and carry to bedside.

Preparation of patient
1. Arrange patient in comfortable position.

Procedure
1. Assemble articles at bedside.
2. Place tub conveniently on bedside table or chair, or in the bed.
3. Arrange a rubber sheet and blanket as a protection for the bed and patient when the tub is placed in the bed.
4. After the arm is in the tub, arrange dressing towel so that edge of tub does not come in contact with arm.
5. Place cover on tub.
Note. — If a foot tub is used, see procedure of hot foot bath.
6. If the bath is continuous, start with a temperature of 105° F. and gradually increase up to 115°. Maintain a temperature of 115° unless otherwise ordered by physician, by adding hot water every 15 minutes. Pour the water into the tub at the extreme corner so as to avoid pouring it on the hand.
7. Prepare fresh solution every 6 hours and scrub and boil the tub once daily, preferably in the morning.

After-care of patient
1. When the treatment is completed, remove arm from tub and dry with a sterile towel.
2. Apply sterile dressings.

After-care of equipment
1. Scrub and boil tub. Replace on shelf.
2. Wash and dry rubber sheet and replace in space provided.
3. Place soiled linen in hamper.

Record
1. In treatment and medication column: time, treatment, kind of solution used, duration.
2. In nurse's remarks column: any observable effects, such as relief of pain, or drainage promoted.
3. Nurse's initials follow all recording.

References
Kelley, *Textbook of Nursing Technique*, p. 246.

Hot Body Pack

Purpose
1. To induce perspiration.
2. To relieve edema.
3. To eliminate waste products.
4. To lower arterial tension.

General instructions
1. Apply cold to head and heat to feet continuously to prevent dilation and congestion of the cerebral blood vessels.
2. Avoid burning patient.
3. Watch for symptoms of heat prostration, such as soft, weak, or irregular pulse, irregular respirations, pallor, or cyanosis.
4. Avoid exposing patient while covers are being removed.
5. Give plenty of fluids, preferably hot, unless liquids are restricted.
6. Work quickly when putting on the steamed blankets. If necessary, use towels for handling.
7. Do not allow wet blankets to come in contact with skin.
8. Do not permit two surfaces of skin to be in contact.
9. Have blankets under patient smooth and free of wrinkles.

Necessary articles
4 wool blankets (1 old thin one).
3 cotton blankets.
Large rubber sheet (mackintosh).
Rubber drawsheet.
Icebag and cover.

Hot-water bag and cover.
Face towel.
Bath towel.
Foot tub or bath basin.
Tray containing a drink, such as lemonade, tea, etc.
Bottle of alcohol for back rub.

Preparation of equipment
1. To prepare the blankets:
   a. Place the rubber mackintosh over the large wool blanket and over it the thin old one.
   b. Fanfold the whole in quarters on both sides to center so that open edge is out.
   c. Fold in half with open edges on inside.
   d. Fold in fourths lengthwise and place on radiator or in warming closet.
   e. Warm third wool blanket also.
   f. Fanfold first cotton blanket in quarters on both sides to center so that open edge is out.
   g. Fanfold second and third cotton blankets end to end in half, then fold back edges to meet in center.
   h. Wet the 3 blankets with hot water and wring as dry as possible.
   i. Place wet blankets over inverted foot tub or basin in tray of utensil sterilizer.
   j. If lid will not close, invert another foot tub over top of sterilizer.
   k. Steam blankets for 20 or 30 minutes.
2. Fill and cover hot-water bottle and icecap.
3. Prepare fluid for patient to drink. When blankets have warmed for required length of time.
   a. Line foot tub with rubber sheet.
   b. Remove blankets from sterilizer and place in tub. Cover with edges of rubber sheet.
   c. Place warmed wool blankets on top.
4. Carry in tub blankets and towels and place on bedside chair.
5. Carry in icecap, hot-water bottle, and fluid for patient.

Preparation of patient
1. Tell patient the nature of the treatment and screen completely.
2. Offer bedpan or allow patient to go to toilet; this may be done while blankets are warming.
3. Remove pillows and place on chair.
4. Fanfold top bedding down and replace with woolen blanket.
5. Place icecap to head and hot-water bottle to feet.

6. Place bath towel over pubic area, remove gown and place over back of chair.
7. Turn patient on side with face away from you.
8. Place warmed woolen blankets and mackintosh under patient with old woolen blanket next to patient.

Procedure

1. Wrap patient well in the old woolen blanket. This is to prevent burning; the wet blankets must not touch the skin.
2. Turn patient on side with face away from you.
3. Place first hot blanket under patient; have her roll back and bring sides up around body.
4. Place second and third blankets on top of patient, tucking in well around body.
5. Bring the mackintosh up around body.
6. Place rubber drawsheet over all and tuck under snugly at sides.
7. Bring up wool blanket on which patient is lying and tuck under smoothly and snugly.
8. Place dry wool blanket over the pack and draw up the covers for added warmth.
9. Place the face towel under patient's chin.
10. Continue pack for as long as ordered. Start timing from the time perspiration starts — 20 minutes is the usual time.
11. Stay with patient all the time she is in the pack.
    a. Take pulse frequently, recording every 15 minutes.
    b. Wipe perspiration from patient's face.
    c. See that icecap is kept in place.
    d. Give drinks at frequent intervals.
    e. Watch for unfavorable symptoms.
12. Remove the pack.
    a. Fanfold covers to foot of bed.
    b. Remove wet blankets and rubber sheets, leaving patient between dry blankets. Do not expose patient while removing the blankets.
13. Remove hot-water bottle.
14. Carry out all equipment.

After-care of patient

1. After 30 minutes or an hour, when perspiration has stopped, give an alcohol rub to the entire body and remove the woolen blanket from under patient.
2. Replace gown; replace wool blanket with covers.
3. Remove screen and leave unit in order.
4. Remove icecap.

After-care of equipment
1. Empty icecap and hot-water bottle; replace.
2. Clean and dry tub and replace.
3. Discard blanket in clothes hamper unless patient is to have pack given again. In that case they are dried, folded, labeled, and put on shelf in linen room.

Record
1. In treatment and medication column: time, treatment, duration, amount of diaphoresis as result.
2. In nurse's remarks column: discomfort or any other unusual reaction as result of treatment.
3. Nurse's initials follow all recording.

References
Harmer, *Principles and Practice of Nursing*, pp. 452–56.
Kelley, *Textbook of Nursing Technique*, pp. 142–44.

IX. GASTRIC EXPRESSIONS AND IRRIGATIONS

Gastric Lavage

Purpose
1. To remove poisons and irritating substances from stomach.
2. To relieve gastric distention.

General instructions
1. When inserting stomach tube, do not use force and avoid striking posterior wall of pharynx.
2. When pouring the fluid, do not allow funnel to become empty.
3. Discontinue the treatment at once if blood appears during the siphonage.
4. All lavages are done by the doctor. The nurse assists the doctor.
5. Be sure tube is in esophagus and not in trachea.

Solutions usually ordered
1. Sodium bicarbonate.
2. Magnesium sulphate.
3. Physiological saline solution.
4. Rainwater.

Temperature of solution
1. 95°–105° F.

Amount of solution
1. 4–8 quarts.

Necessary articles

Face towel.	Funnel.
Rubber sheet.	Pulitzer bulb.
Safety pin.	Solution.
Small rubber square or newspaper.	Pail or foot tub.
Stomach tube in basin of chipped ice.	Tray.

Preparation of equipment
1. Boil stomach tube, bulb, and funnel 3 minutes. Remove and place in basin of chipped ice.
2. Arrange other articles on tray.
3. Carry tray and pail or tub to bedside.

Preparation of patient
1. Explain nature of treatment to patient and screen completely.
2. Have patient sitting in chair or in semi-recumbent position in bed.
3. Pin towel and rubber sheet around patient's neck.

4. Place rubber or newspaper on chair, and pail or tub on chair beside bed.

Procedure

1. The doctor inserts the tube gently, instructing the patient to breathe deeply through her mouth and to swallow frequently.
2. The tube is usually inserted to the graduated mark, or about 16 inches.
3. The solution is poured into the funnel, which is held not more than 6 inches above patient's head. About a pint is poured in at once. The tube is then lowered over the tub and the contents siphoned off. If necessary, the funnel can be removed and the contents expressed by means of the bulb.
4. Repeat until the solution returns clear.
5. In withdrawing tube see that it is pinched tightly to prevent aspiration of solution into the lungs.

After-care of patient
1. If bed has been soiled, put on clean linen.
2. See that patient is comfortable.

After-care of equipment
1. Clean tube, bulb, and funnel by flushing several times with cold water.
2. Boil 3 minutes, remove, dip in cold water, dry, and replace.
3. Wash rubber sheet with soap and water, if necessary, dry, and replace.
4. Scour, wash, and dry tub; replace.

Record
1. In treatment and medication column: time, treatment, kind and amount of solution, by whom given, character and amount of return flow.
2. In nurse's remarks column: any abnormalities noted, comfort resulting or discomfort during or after treatment.
3. Nurse's initials follow all recording.

References
Harmer, *Principles and Practice of Nursing*, pp. 475–81.
Kelley, *Textbook of Nursing Technique*, pp. 213–15.

Fractional Gastric Expression

Purpose
1. To determine the amount of free hydrochloric acid in the stomach after stimulation.

General instructions
1. The patient should have had no food for at least 4 hours before test.

2. Give food or other liquids only as ordered by doctor until the test is complete.
3. Sometimes changing position or having patient swallow a bit more tube will facilitate securing the contents.

Stimulants used
1. Ewald test meal:
   a. 2 slices of one-day-old bread without crust or 2 slices of toast.
   b. 1 or 2 glasses of water or cups of tea.
   c. Bowl of cooked cereal.
2. Alcohol:
   a. Strength and amount depending upon doctor in charge of department.
3. Histamine (ergomine) order for dosage written before each administration, usually from 0.25–0.5 milligrams.

Necessary articles
Tray.
Duodenal tube or nasal catheter.
20 cc. Luer syringe.
40 cc. test tubes, number depending upon the number of specimens routinely taken.
Gummed labels.
Paper clip.
Kidney basin.
Topfer's solution.
Small rubber square.
Face towel.

Preparation of equipment
1. Cover tray with unsterile towel.
2. Boil duodenal tube 3 minutes and place in dressing bowl filled with chipped ice.
3. Label tubes with numbered gummed labels; place upright in container.
4. Arrange other articles on tray and carry to bedside.

Preparation of patient
1. Tell patient the nature of the test and the importance of co-operation.
2. Screen completely.
3. Make comfortable in a semi-recumbent position.
4. Place rubber square covered with a face towel around neck and pin in place.

Procedure
1. Assist doctor as necessary in helping patient swallow the tube.

2. Obtain 10 cc. of fasting content by aspirating with syringe. Expel from syringe into test tube no. 1.
3. Give stimulant.
4. Aspirate desired number of specimens at 15-minute intervals. Effort should be made to obtain 10 cc. for each specimen. Use test tubes in order of marking.
5. Between specimens compress tube close to mouth with paper clip to prevent drainage of contents from end of tube.
6. Following expression of last specimen notify head nurse so that if desired the specimens may be tested for free hydrochloric acid with Topfer's solution in station laboratory. (Upon the addition of a few drops of the dye the specimen becomes bright red in color if it contains free hydrochloric acid.)
7. If in absence of free hydrochloric acid in first specimens histamine is ordered, administer hypodermically.
8. Aspirate desired number of specimens at 15-minute intervals.
9. Watch patient carefully during half hour following injection of histamine for symptoms of toxicity — headache, increased pulse rate, flushed face, etc.
10. When test is finished, pinch off tube and withdraw gently, but quickly.
11. Remove towel from around neck and leave patient comfortable.

After-care of patient
1. If patient has had tray withheld, warm food and serve.

After-care of equipment
1. Send specimen to laboratory with request blank.
2. Wash duodenal tube well, boil 3 minutes, rinse in cold water, and put away.
3. Clean other articles used and replace.

Record
1. In treatment column: time, treatment, stimulant used, number of specimens collected, time of collection, specimens to laboratory.
2. In nurse's remarks column: any difficulty in passing tube or obtaining specimen.
3. Nurse's initials follow all recording.

References
Harmer, *Principles and Practice of Nursing*, pp. 483–89.
Kelley, *Textbook of Nursing Technique*, pp. 215–17.

Nasal Suction

Purpose
1. To relieve distention in the stomach and duodenum by the removal of gas.
2. To afford a frequent lavage of the stomach to remove irritating and nauseating material.

General instructions
1. Amount of fluid is measured only when so ordered by the doctor.
2. The suction is not to be turned off for any length of time except by doctor's order.
3. Suction will be furnished in the duodenal tube as long as there is any fluid in the upper bottle.
4. Gas entering the upper bottle causes it to become empty.

Necessary articles
From Sterile Supply Room:
Autoclaved tray with:
Nasal catheter.
2 pieces of rubber tubing with screw clamps, one 6 feet long and the other 4 feet with glass connector.
2-holed rubber stopper with 2 glass tubes run through it, 1 tube 4 inches long, the other 14 inches.
Brass screw for top of bottle.
2 gallon glass bottles.
Metal holder and handle for gallon bottle.
Irrigation standard.
Medicine glass.
Adhesive ½ inch wide.

Preparation of equipment
1. Open tray and place on it medicine glass half full of mineral oil.
2. Fill 1 gallon bottle full of tap water.
3. Remove stopper from tray and put in bottle. Screw down brass top to hold stopper in place.
4. Put 400 cc. tap water in second bottle.
5. Carry all articles to bedside. Place irrigation standard at the head of bed.

Preparation of patient
1. Explain to patient what the treatment is to be and what relief he will obtain from it.
2. Screen patient while the procedure is being started. He need not be screened all the time it is being given.

Procedure

1. The physician lubricates the nasal catheter and inserts it through the nose and into the stomach or duodenum. Have water and a glass tube there so that patient may drink while tube is being passed.
2. The nurse attaches the rubber tubing to the glass tubes in the stopper, the longest tubing being attached to the shortest glass tube and the shortest tubing to the longest glass tube.
3. Clamp off both tubes.
4. Place bottle in holder and hang up on standard, 6 feet above the floor.
5. Place other bottle on the floor below.
6. Put longest rubber tube, i. e., the one from the shortest glass tube, into the floor bottle.
7. Remove clamp from longest rubber tube; then, with the finger over the tip of the other tube, remove the clamp on that also. Suction should immediately be perceived by the fingertip. As soon as it is, clamp off both tubes. (If suction is not felt only one thing can be the cause — air in the tube. Look at stopper in top bottle to be sure that it is tight, then look at the end of tube in the floor bottle and make sure that the end is covered by the water. Then if suction is not felt, inject a few cubic centimeters of tap water with a syringe into the tube connected to the longer glass tube.)
8. As soon as suction is felt, the tubes are clamped off and the nasal tube is attached to the tube leading to the longest glass tube.
9. The nasal tube is fastened to the face with a piece of adhesive.
10. Unclamp both tubes to their full extent, but leave clamps there for future use.
11. The length of time that the suction is to be continued depends on the doctor's order.

After-care of patient

1. As a rule the patient may have as much water as he desires.
2. No milk nor any solid food may be given because that will stop up the tubes.
3. Once a day inject 1 medicine dropperful of argyrol 2 per cent in the nose along the outside of the tube. Alboline may be substituted if the patient prefers.
4. Report any discomfort to the nose or throat to the interne; he will usually change the tube to the opposite side of the nose to avoid undue irritation.
5. Observe closely and report any distention or nausea that may occur when suction is shut off.

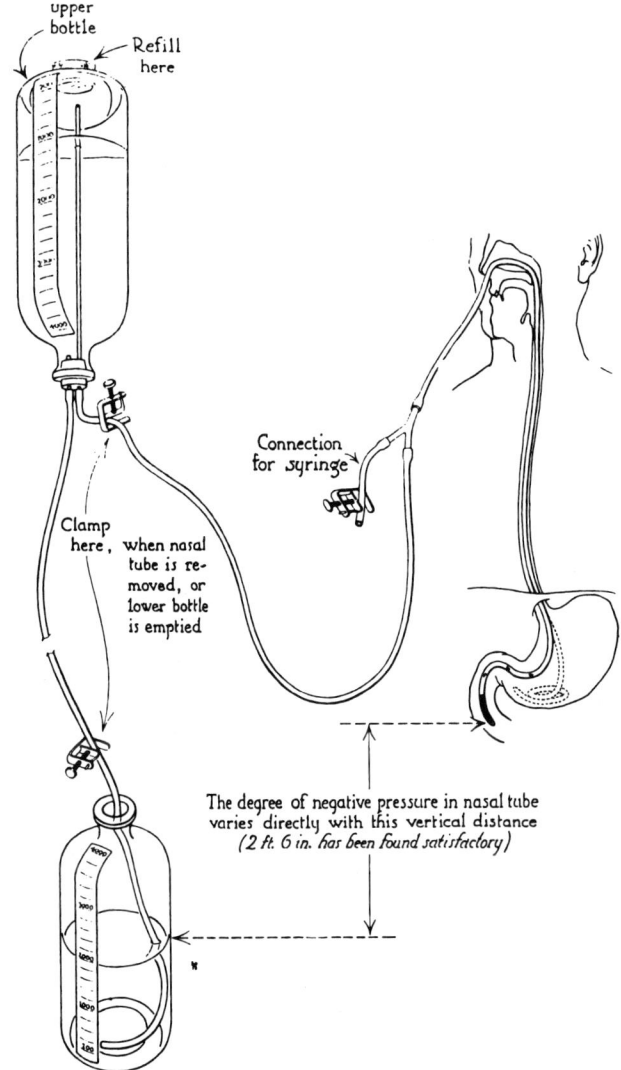

The degree of negative pressure in nasal tube
varies directly with this vertical distance
(2 ft. 6 in. has been found satisfactory)

After-care of equipment

1. While suction is running:
   a. Prevent lower bottle from running over when patient drinks large amounts of fluid.
   b. Change and restart bottles according to hospital routine.
   c. If upper bottle empties too quickly, there is air in the set-up. Inspect tubing and connections for leaks.
   d. If nasal tube becomes plugged with mucus or because patient has taken something by mouth other than strained

clear liquids, undo the nasal catheter at the glass connection tube, inject 5–10 cc. of drinking water with a syringe, and then draw it back into the syringe; repeat until tube is free. Be sure you remove all that you inject or the total fluid intake of the patient will not be accurate.

2. After the suction has been discontinued:
   a. Wash rubber tubing under force and boil 5 minutes.
   b. Wash both bottles with tap water. If they are at all incrusted, use an alkali, such as sodium bicarbonate or tr. green soap, to remove the acid crusts. Then boil the bottles 5 minutes.

3. Return equipment to Sterile Supply Room in good order.

Record

1. In treatment and medication column:
   When amount taken is ordered:
   a. When treatment is started: time, treatment, by whom, amount in upper bottle, amount in lower bottle.
   b. When bottles are refilled: time, amount emptied from each bottle, amount refilled in each bottle.
   c. When treatment is discontinued: time discontinued, amount in each bottle.
   When not necessary to measure amount: time, treatment, by whom, time discontinued.

2. In nurse's remarks column: relief from nausea and distention, or discomfort caused by treatment.

3. On fluid record: night nurse calculates amount absorbed and adds to oral intake.

Note. — To calculate the retention or absorption: total amount in bottles at start and added later + total amount taken by mouth = total intake. Total amount emptied from bottles = total output. Total intake — total output = total absorption.

References

Paine and Phillips, "Nasal Catheter Suction: Siphonage," *American Journal of Nursing*, 1933, pp. 525–33.

Oral Gavage

Purpose

1. To introduce food into stomach when patient cannot or will not take food in the normal manner.

Solution used

1. Concentrated, nourishing liquid food as ordered.

Temperature of solution

100°–105° F.

Quantity of solution
4–10 ounces.

Necessary articles
Face towel.
Rubber sheet.
Safety pin.
Small rubber square or newspaper.
Stomach tube in basin of chipped ice.
Funnel.
Solution.
Graduate containing prepared food.
Tray.

Preparation of equipment
1. Boil stomach tube and funnel 3 minutes, remove, and place in basin of chipped ice.
2. Prepare kind and quantity of food as ordered.
3. Arrange all articles on tray and carry to bedside.

Preparation of patient
1. Explain nature of treatment to patient and screen completely.
2. Have patient sitting in chair or semi-recumbent position in bed.
3. Pin towel and rubber sheet around patient's neck.

Procedure
1. The doctor inserts the tube gently, instructing the patient to breathe deeply through the mouth and to swallow frequently.
2. The tube is usually inserted to the graduated mark, or about 16 inches.
3. The funnel is elevated about 6 inches above patient's head and the solution poured into it.
4. Pour solution down the side of funnel until tube is filled in order to prevent forcing air into stomach.
5. When all the solution has been given, pinch the tube tightly and withdraw it gently but quickly.

After-care of patient
1. If bed has become soiled, put on clean linen.
2. See that patient is comfortable.

After-care of equipment
1. Clean tube and funnel by flushing several times with cold water.
2. Boil 3 minutes, remove, dip in cold water, dry, and replace.
3. Give care to rubber sheet if necessary.
4. Clean and replace other articles used.

Record

1. In treatment and medication column: time, kind, amount given, treatment, by whom.
2. In nurse's remarks column: any difficulty in passing tube or other reaction the patient may have.
3. Nurse's initials follow all recording.

References

Harmer, *Principles and Practice of Nursing*, pp. 481–82.
Kelley, *Textbook of Nursing Technique,* pp. 219–20.

Nasal Gavage

Purpose

1. To introduce food into the stomach:
   a. When patient is very weak.
   b. When cooperation of patient is impossible.
   c. When there is danger of patient biting tube.
   d. When abnormal condition of jaws or mouth contra-indicates passing tube by mouth.

General instructions

1. Be sure that the catheter is in the esophagus and not in the mouth, larynx, or trachea.
2. Watch breathing and color of patient while inserting the tube.
3. By placing free end of catheter below surface of solution and watching for bubble, make sure the tube is in the esophagus and not in the larynx.
4. If obstruction is met, withdraw the tube and insert in the other nostril.

Solution used

1. Concentrated, nourishing liquid food, as ordered.

Temperature of solution

100°–105° F.

Quantity of solution

4–10 ounces.

Necessary articles

Face towel. (That at patient's bedside may be used.)
Safety pin.
Nasal catheter in solution basin.
Mineral oil, 4 drams in medicine glass.
Triumph syringe or small funnel.
Kidney basin.
Graduate containing prepared food.
Tray.

Preparation of equipment
1. Boil tube, syringe, solution basin, and kidney basin 3 minutes.
2. Remove from boiler and place tube in dressing bowl and syringe in kidney basin.
3. Prepare kind and quantity of food as ordered.
4. Arrange all articles on tray and carry to bedside.

Preparation of patient
1. Explain nature of treatment to patient and screen completely.
2. Have patient sitting in chair or semi-recumbent position in bed.
3. Have patient lying down with head turned to one side or sitting up with head tilted forward.

Procedure
1. Lubricate, then insert catheter, directing toward the septum of the nose so that about 4 inches is passed into the esophagus.
2. Wait until normal breathing is established before pouring in the liquid.
3. Pour in only a few drops at first; if no coughing follows, you may feel quite certain the tube is in the esophagus.
4. When all the fluid has left the funnel, pinch the catheter and withdraw gently but quickly.
5. If feeding is to be repeated at frequent intervals, the tube may be clamped off and fastened to patient's gown between feedings.

After-care of patient
1. If bed has become soiled, put on clean linen.
2. See that patient is comfortable.

After-care of equipment
1. Flush tube several times with cold water, boil 3 minutes, dip in cold water, dry, and replace.
2. Give care to other articles used.

Record
1. In treatment and medication column: time, kind, amount given, treatment, by whom.
2. In nurse's remarks column: any difficulty in passing the tube or other reaction the patient may have.
3. Nurse's initials follow all recording.

References
Harmer, *Principles and Practice of Nursing*, pp. 482–83.
Kelley, *Textbook of Nursing Technique*, pp. 220–21.

X. THE CARE OF THE DEAD

Purpose
1. To have the body straight and clean and in proper condition for the morgue.
2. To avoid causing discoloration of face or hands.

General instructions
1. If possible, patients in terminal conditions are moved from the ward into a room.
2. When patients are left in the ward they should be well screened.
3. Care should be given the body as soon as the doctor has pronounced the patient dead.
4. Avoid unnecessary exposure.
5. The body should be moved as little as possible after death and never placed face downward.
6. Treat the body with reverence; remember that "the body is the temple of the soul."
7. A nurse must remain at the bedside of a dying patient.
8. Note exact time patient ceases to breathe.
9. Arrange body in suitable position before rigor mortis sets in.
10. Notify immediately those who are to be told of death.
11. Care for clothing and valuables according to routine of hospital.

Necessary articles
Morgue roll containing:
  Morgue sheet.
  Large cellu-cotton pad.
  3-inch bandage.
  2 clothes tags.
  3 safety pins.
  Paper bag.
  4 safety pins (for pinning roll).
Bath and toilet articles.
If patient has dressing on:
  Carbon tetrachloride or other solvent for adhesive.
  Abdominal pad.
  Adhesive.
Envelope for jewelry.

Preparation of equipment
1. Secure morgue roll from Sterile Supply Room.
2. Open, check contents, and make out cards with patient's

name, age, registry number, date and hour of death, name of nurse or orderly in attendance.

3. If patient has no comb or nail file, secure these.
4. If material for putting on clean dressings is indicated, secure these also.
5. Place all articles in morgue basket.
6. Carry to bedside.
7. Carry basin of water to bedside.

Preparation of patient

1. As soon as doctor has pronounced patient dead and members of family have left room, straighten limbs.
2. Close the eyes naturally — they will usually stay closed if held with the finger tips for a few seconds.
3. Leave 2 pillows under the head; remove all others.
4. If patient has false teeth, put them in the mouth at once and close the mouth by means of a rolled towel placed under the chin.
5. Straighten covers and cover face with upper sheet.
6. This preparation is given the body before the equipment is prepared.

Procedure

1. Remove all jewelry, place in envelope, and care for it afterwards according to routine of hospital.
2. Remove all covers except top sheet.
3. Remove gown.
4. Replace dressings (if any) with fresh ones. Remove unattached drainage tubes, artery clamps, splints, etc. Adhesive marks should be removed.
5. Bathe face and anterior of body with soap and water.
6. Turn on side, bathe back; while body is turned on side, adjust morgue sheet so that one corner is at head and one at feet; also place pad under buttocks.
7. Comb hair and care for the nails.
8. Leave arms at sides of body.
9. Loosely attach one of the tags to one wrist with string.
10. Remove towel from under chin; bring corner of sheet down over face, and sides of sheet up; pin with one safety pin so that sheet is loose about face but tight enough around jaws to give some support. Be sure that ears are in natural position.
11. Pin sheet together in center of body with 4 safety pins with which morgue roll was pinned.
12. The second tag is pinned outside the sheet over the chest.

After-care of body

1. Call an orderly.

2. Place body on stretcher carefully and gently and cover with sheet and blanket.
3. Before bringing body into the hall, see that elevator is at floor and that no patients are in the hall.
4. An orderly usually takes the body to the morgue, but a nurse must accompany him.
5. The body is placed in the vault in the morgue with head elevated.
6. Routine reports:
   a. University Hospital:
      (1) Triplicate death notices; one is sent to the School of Nursing Office, one goes with the body, and one to the superintendent of the hospital.
      (2) Put name, hour of death, and service on census slip.
      (3) Remove card from diet chart and cross off name on defecation chart.
   b. Miller Hospital:
      (1) Same as 2 and 3 under University Hospital.
      (2) Three notification slips are made out by head nurse; one is sent to superintendent of hospital, one to the superintendent of nurses, and one to the main office.
      (3) See that the pathologist is notified.
      (4) Cross off name on daily report sheet.
      (5) White stockings and gown are put on, and chin brace must be used.
      (6) A charge slip is made out for gown, large pad, sheet, and stockings. Patient may use own, if available.
   c. Minneapolis General Hospital:
      (1) Take patient's name from census board.
      (2) Place body in a compartment in the morgue and insert name slip in holder on door.
      (3) Fill out morgue sheet with patient's name, date, and hour put in morgue.
      (4) Triplicate death notices are sent out, two to information desk and one to School of Nursing Office.

After-care of equipment
1. Replace morgue basket and other articles used.
2. Strip bed and give care to unit as after discharge of patient.
3. Care of patient's belongings:
   a. All rings, earrings, bracelets, beads, and emblems of sacred or religious significance should be removed, listed, and placed in the envelope with other articles of value, such as money, receipts, eye glasses, letters, keys, etc. At top of list write patient's name and registry number and take to

Business Office, if in daytime. If at night, put in a secure place and notify head nurse in the morning.

b. All clothing and other personal property should be checked, neatly wrapped in a bundle, properly tagged, and taken to the Property Room, or handled according to routine of hospital.

c. If relatives wish to take valuables or personal belongings of deceased from the station, make a complete list and have them sign statement that they have taken them.

Record

1. In nurse's remarks column: hour of death, by whom certified, anything unusual connected with death.

References

Harmer, *Principles and Practice of Nursing*, pp. 367–70.

Kelley, *Textbook of Nursing Technique*, pp. 137–38.

XI. SPECIAL PROCEDURES FOR THE COMMUNICABLE DISEASE DEPARTMENT

Theory of Aseptic Technique

General principles

The theory of aseptic technique is based on the fact that infections are transmitted by actual contact, direct and indirect.

Indirect contact takes place through a contaminated carrier. Air transmission is rare and is therefore not considered of particular importance, except that the doors of rooms occupied by measles, chicken-pox, and smallpox patients are always kept closed. The nurse must be careful, however, not to allow the patient to cough in her face.

Anything that has come directly or indirectly in contact with patients or any infected area is contaminated.

A room or ward occupied by one or more patients representing a separate and distinct infection constitutes a unit. Everything within the unit is considered contaminated. See further discussion of this point under "The unit," page 221.

The aim is to confine each different infection to a separate unit and to prevent the transmission of infection from one unit to another. All areas on the stations not included in units, such as corridors, linen closets, kitchens, etc., are clean.

Gowns supplied for the purpose are worn while treating patients and while cleaning in the unit. Care is taken not to contaminate the inner clean side of the gown. After the treatment has been given, the hands are washed in the hand solution or in soap and water. The gown is removed and folded so as to cover the inside. It is hung on a hook in the unit so that it may be used again. The hands are scrubbed before treating other patients.

New patients are kept under observation after admission and treated in units of one until two or more reports of nose and throat cultures are received. If these prove satisfactory, the patients are moved into wards if this type of isolation is employed.

All floors in contagious and isolation stations are considered contaminated.

The nurse must remember:

1. To wash her hands frequently and always before eating.
2. Not to touch her face nor anything clean when her hands are contaminated.
3. Not to allow children to touch her face.
4. To eat nothing a patient has handled and not to partake of food in a patient's room.

5. To wear a mask when on duty in the contagious section and to wear it over the mouth and nose when caring for patients.
6. To take some out-of-door exercise every day.
7. To sleep with windows open.
8. To take a bath daily.
9. If indisposed, to report at once to the nurse in charge.
10. Not to share a room with anyone who is ill.
11. To have nose and throat cultures for diphtheria once a week.
12. Always to call a person's attention to a breach of technique.
13. To stay away from the stations when off duty.
14. That sleeves of long gowns must not be rolled.
15. That contaminated articles must not be placed in waste baskets but burned in the incinerators.
16. That contaminated linen is not to be placed on the floor, but in hampers for the purpose.
17. That paper sacks are to be used in all patients' rooms.
18. That isolation gowns are not to be worn in the corridor.
19. That students must have nose and throat cultures taken on the day previous to leaving the contagious service.

The unit
A unit is "a sharply defined zone of contamination." — Stimson. It includes the patient and his immediate surroundings, such as his bed, bedside table, chair, utensils if kept in the unit and not sterilized every time used, thermometer, etc. Actually anything contaminated by the patient is part of the unit until disposed of. This includes the waste being carried from the unit to the incinerator, etc.
"Sharply defined" may mean:
1. The four walls of a room. Everything in the unit is considered contaminated except the electric-light buttons.
2. The glass cubicle partitions. These partitions are found in wards. The rest of the ward unoccupied by patients must be kept clean.
3. Imaginary lines. The rest of ward remains clean.
On the stations for the highly contagious diseases, each patient is in an individual unit. On the isolation station where are the diseases not so readily communicable, a unit may consist of more than one patient, all having the same disease. The first type of isolation is the patient-unit system, the latter is the disease-unit system.

Admission of Patients

Preparation of the room:
1. Select from the available rooms the one that will best satisfy the patient's condition, i. e., steam room for laryngeal cases —

steam may not be used, but often it is; quiet room for meningitis cases, etc.

2. The room should contain only the articles necessary for the care of the patient.
3. Make up foundation of bed only.
4. Equip room with bathtub, wash basin, bedpan, emesis basin, mouthwash cup, face and bath towels, washcloth, soap in soap dish, toilet paper, and paper bag.
5. Thermometer in cup of solution of bichloride of mercury 1/1000 is placed on shelf.
6. If thermometer is to be a rectal thermometer, also place lubricant-petrolatum on the shelf.
7. Gown on hook.
8. Solution of disinfectant in hand solution basin.
9. Remove table and chair from side of bed so they will be out of the way when the patient is wheeled in.
10. The door of the room is left open.

General instructions

1. Patients for the contagious service are admitted directly to the Receiving Department in the Annex Building. When a patient is to be admitted, the nurse or clerk at the Annex Office Desk will call Station M, notifying the station of the patient's presence in the admitting room. A nurse from the station goes to the Receiving Department to admit the patient.
2. Be sure your mask covers your mouth and nose. Wear a gown when the procedure makes it necessary.
3. The patient usually is on a stretcher, having been placed there by the ambulance driver. He is, in this case, undressed, having on a hospital gown.
4. The patient may be sitting on the chair, fully clothed, having come in from the main Receiving Department.
5. The patient may be a child, accompanied by the mother or some other adult.

Procedure (The order may vary according to the case.)

1. Assist the patient to undress and help him on to the stretcher. When a mother accompanies a child, she may undress him and put him on the stretcher.
2. Take the temperature, pulse, and respiration.
3. Make the patient as comfortable as possible.
4. Scrub the hands for 2 minutes.
5. When clean, fill out admission card. Every item is to be filled in. If information for some item is not available, draw a line through the space, indicating that you have considered it.

6. Assist doctor in taking nose and throat cultures.
7. Assist doctor while he examines the patient.
8. Consent sheets:
   When the doctor wishes permission to perform spinal punctures, myringotomies, etc., on a patient too young to sign for himself, if the parent is with the child, have this parent sign the consent *under isolation technique*. The relatives and friends are considered contaminated to the patient.
9. When the above procedures have been executed, cover the patient as taught and take to a room on the station. See that he is comfortable. Now would be, routinely, the time for the admission bath, but it will be necessary to return to the Annex Office with the stretcher and finish the admission routine. Report to nurse in charge that patient is on the station.
10. Clean any part of the admission room that has become contaminated.
11. Set up Admission Room. See that cupboard is in order.
12. Take cultures, culture slip, and admission card to the Annex Office. The nurse or clerk will take care of the cultures and will make out the chart.
13. Call the main Receiving Department for a case number. This is written on the admission card, the property book, the chart, and the tag on the clothing bag.
14. Leave the admission card at the Annex Office desk; the nurse or clerk will take it to the Receiving Department. She also has charge of registering the patient's name in the admission book, etc.
15. Return to station.
16. Give patient bedside care according to the admission routine.

Care of belongings

1. If a patient has clothing and valuables with him and if one of the family accompanies the patient, put clothing and valuables in a clean paper bag and let the relative take these articles home. (Make a cuff on your bag so you can close it without contaminating your hands.) Instruct the family how to clean the articles. The clothes may be taken home because the family and the house from which the patient came are considered contaminated.
   Register the name in the "Ledger Property Book." State that clothing and valuables were taken home. Record the date. Later record the case number. Sign your name and have the patient or a member of the family sign the book. This is done under isolation technique, as taught, for the signing of clean documents by contaminated patients.

2. If the patient comes alone and has clothing and valuables, list clothing and valuables in the itemized clothing book and have the patient sign the book without contaminating it. The nurse signs as witness. Put clothing in hamper bag, keeping outside clean, as taught. The blue property slip goes inside the bag (after the case number has been written on the sheet). On the outside, at the top edge, pin a red contaminated tag and a small white tag on which is written the patient's name, case number, date, and "To the property room after hotboxing." The valuables, such as money, keys, etc., are scrubbed with soap and water and placed in special envelopes (the clothing list is printed on the outside). The pink property list goes in this envelope. Be sure the case number is on the slip. Take this envelope and the property book to the business office; one of the clerks will check the valuables with you and o. k. the book. The valuables are retained in the business office until the patient is discharged.

3. If the patient has no clothes and no valuables, write his name and date in the "Ledger Property Book." Also write, "No clothing or valuables." Have the patient sign the book under isolation technique. The nurse signs as witness.

4. If the patient is unconscious or for any other reason cannot sign, make the necessary notations as indicated above. Sign the book and have some other nurse sign also.

Routine for Annex Receiving Department

A nurse from Station M is responsible for the care of the Receiving Department. A nurse is usually assigned this duty for one week. She takes care of this unit immediately after morning circle. In addition, she is responsible for the nurse's dressing room.

Care of admitting unit

1. Check supplies in admitting rooms:
   a. On the table:
      (1) Top
         (a) Forms: admission cards, history sheets, physical sheets, operation permits, etc.
         (b) Culture tubes, sterile applicators, tongue depressors, culture slips. Keep inside a doctor's towel. The materials are obtained from the Annex Office.
         (c) Ink, pen, pencil, and blotter.
      (2) Lower shelf:
         (a) A mask within a clean doctor's towel.
         (b) Paper toweling.

b. Change the disinfectant in the brush basin daily. Measure water and disinfectant accurately.

c. See that an isolation gown is hanging, as taught, on the hook in admitting room.

d. See that the stretcher is draped as taught.

e. The paper bags in the waste paper stand are to be changed daily.

Note. — Into a clean paper bag that has an external cuff made on it, place the contaminated bags. Scrub for 2 minutes. (The refuse sometimes drops outside the bag. The refuse is, as a rule, contaminated.) Clean the frame baskets with disinfectant. Place clean bags in each frame basket. When you return to the station, take the clean bag containing the contaminated ones with you. Burn it in incinerator.

f. See that the entire unit is scrupulously clean.

2. Check supplies in metal cupboards:

a. Check drugs, thermometers, supplies, etc. Do not let any set of supplies become wholly exhausted. Replenish before the last is used. This will save the embarrassment that comes from lack of equipment and it will aid you in knowing what to order.

b. Check linen, such as sheets, blankets, etc.

Check nurses' caps, belts, gowns, and masks. Check gowns according to size: M, medium; S, small; L, large. This letter is found on the inside of the neck. Make out a list of linen needed. If you have been taught to do this in the linen book, do so. Otherwise take a detailed list with actual number of articles needed to the nurse in charge of Station M.

c. Make blanket rolls. Each of these includes three *large* blankets, one sheet, and one patient's gown.

Note. — Use large blankets only. These are folded lengthwise, separately, as demonstrated, the one placed upon the other after being folded. The sheet and patient's gown are rolled within the blanket and the roll is pinned and tagged according to the size of gown within, i. e., large, medium, small.

Important. — If the large-size patient's gown seems too short to cover the patient well, it will be necessary to use a long isolation gown. Keep 9 blanket rolls on hand, 3 of each size.

d. Look through the clothing book to see if any valuables have been collected since 5 P. M. of the day preceding. If any have been collected after 8:30 A. M., take the clothing book to the business office and check these valuables with the business office. The envelope containing the valuables is on file in this office.

e. Arrange cupboard neatly.

f. Tie up hamper bag, mark with red contaminated tag. It will be collected and taken to laundry. Leave it near elevator. Place a clean hamper bag on the hamper standard.

g. Lock doors and return keys to Annex Office.

h. Take hamper bags, etc., and go to nurses' dressing room.

Ward care of newly admitted patients

1. Enter unit, greet patient, make him by your attitude and greeting feel as comfortable, mentally and spiritually, as you can.

2. Put on gown.

3. Take temperature, pulse, and respiration.

4. Since the diagnosis has been made in the admitting room and the patient has therefore been examined by a doctor, an admission bath may be given.

5. Note symptoms.

6. Make up the bed and make the patient as comfortable as possible.

7. Carry out any orders there may be for your patient.

8. Leave on the bedside table, within easy reach of the patient, a pitcher of drinking water and a glass drinking tube if the doctor has already ordered it.

9. Give instructions to patient:

   a. Patient must not sit up or get out of bed without the doctor's permission.

   b. The floor is contaminated and patient must not pick up anything from the floor.

10. Remove gown.

11. Scrub for 2 minutes.

12. Chart.

Care of Patients

Gown Technique

To put on gown

1. Enter unit. Do not touch anything.
2. Palms together, put hands through opening in gown, letting fingertips come to the shoulder seams (Figure A). (The fingertips guide the sleeves so that they will not swing back and contaminate the uniform). Let thumbs drop back to outer corners of neckband. Using the elbows to further open the back of gown, slip on the gown. By using thumbs and elbows as above directed you can guide the back of the gown so that the outside will not turn in and contaminate the uniform. Do not let hands touch outside of gown.
3. Place forefinger of each hand within neckband in front. Follow neckband to the back (Figure B). Grasp strings. Tie strings. (Sleeves must not come in contact with back of head or with the cap.)
4. Grasp left string at seam with little finger of left hand. Grasp right string at seam with little finger of right hand (Figure C). Bring both forward and hold both strings with little finger of left hand (Figure D). (The other fingers of left hand are kept clean to later grasp clean left side.) Grasp with free right hand the back edge of right side of gown. Bringing this forward, take from the left hand the strings of the grown. With free left hand (remember the little finger is contaminated) grasp back edge of left side still holding the sides of the gown, drop the strings (Figure E). Cross gown in back, putting left side underneath always. Sleeve is contaminated, so must not touch gown (Figures F and G.) If left side of the gown becomes contaminated, it will contaminate the inside of the right side when the right side is crossed over the left in back (Figure H). Bring strings forward. Tie in front (Figure I).
5. Pull up sleeves so the cuffs will not slip down during the procedure you are to execute. If they do, the gown is discarded at the end of the procedure.
6. The gown, though considered contaminated, should be kept free from contamination from six inches below shoulders upward.

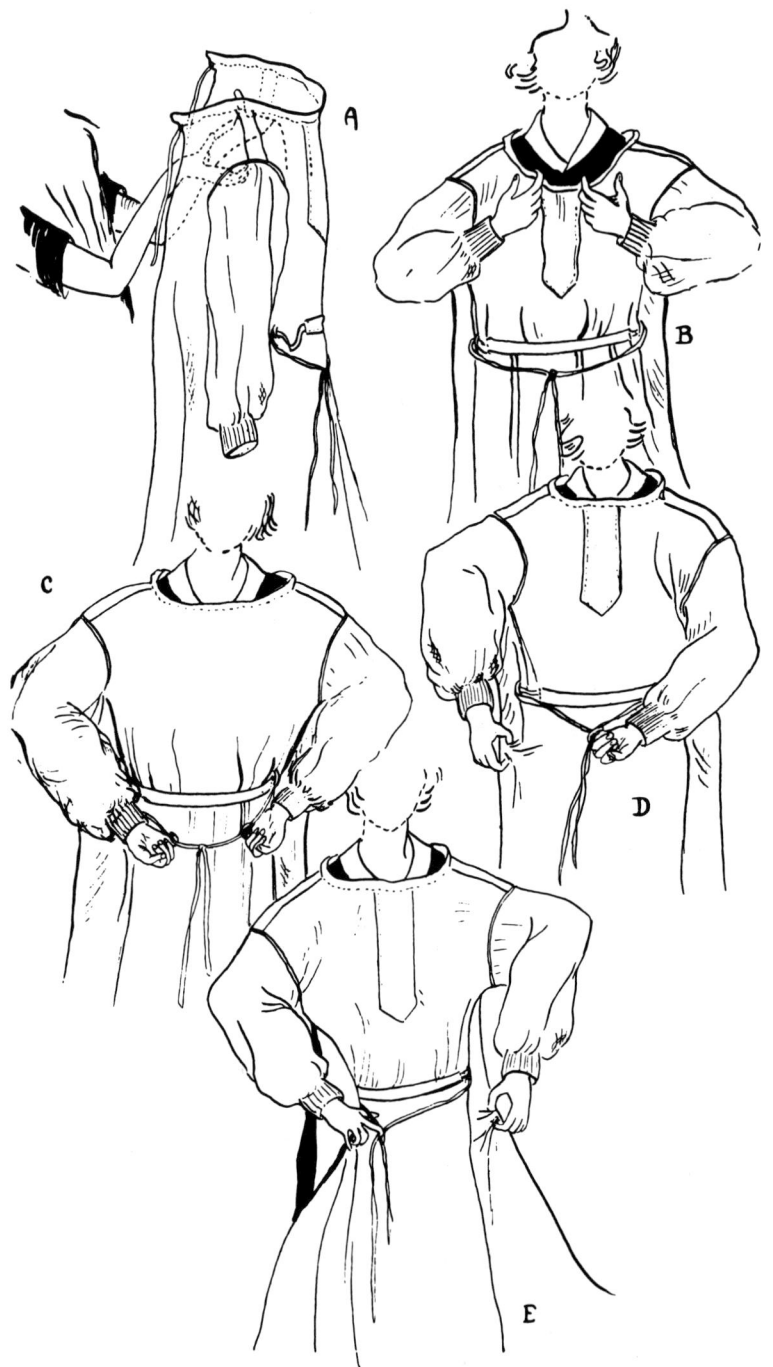

The sketches on this and the following page illustrate the
technique of putting on the gown.

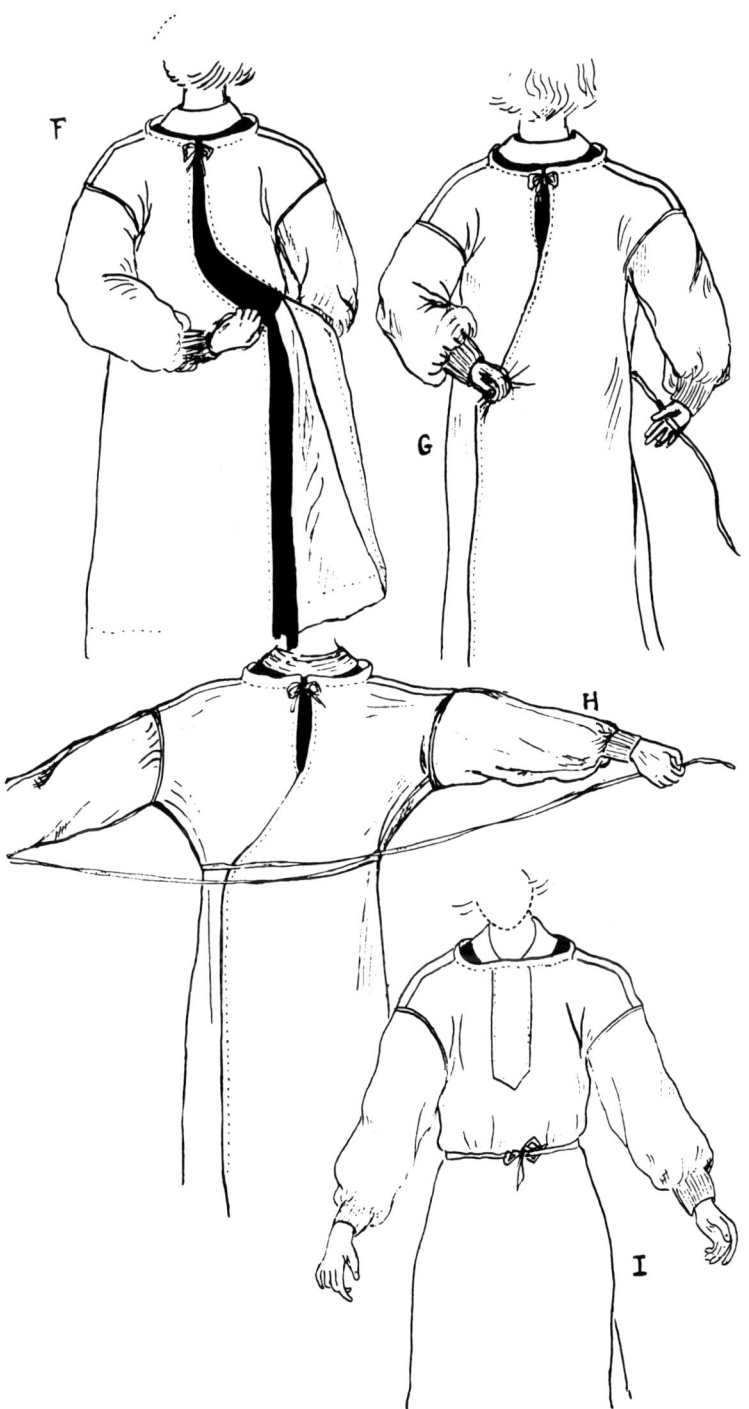

See page 227 for an explanation of the technique
of putting on the gown.

To remove gown
1. Untie strings at waist, bring forward, and loop them in front (Figure A).
2. Pull sleeves up about an inch (Figure A).
3. Wash the hands to about ½ inch from edge of sleeve. (Note: If the arms are washed up to the cuff, as would ordinarily be the case if entire arm below cuff is contaminated, the hands will still be contaminated, having touched a contaminated sleeve. If, however, there is a clean margin between contaminated part of arm and sleeve edge, recontamination of hands will be avoided.)
4. Untie strings at neck, letting them hang down center of back (Figure A). Come out of sleeve as follows: Place forefinger of right hand under cuff of left sleeve and pull down over hand (Figures B and C). Keep hands clean. Do not touch outside of gown. Through sleeve of left hand, the left hand grasps the outer part of right cuff and works it off over right hand (Figure D). Continue to come out of gown, working hand up to neck and bringing two ends of neckband together. Grasp back of gown, including strings in one hand and front of gown in other (Figure E). (Grasp from back and from front. *Never over* edge of neck.) Fanfold shoulder seams up toward neck, hang by shoulder seams. The neckband and strings must be against wall (that above the hook is clean) and not hanging down against sleeve (Figure F).
6. You are now considered contaminated.
7. Scrub in outer, clean scrub room for two minutes.

"Scrubbing" Technique

CARE OF HANDS OUTSIDE UNIT

This procedure is necessary to remove all infective material from nurse's hands before she cares for any other patient or any other articles outside of the unit she has just left.

Necessary articles
Basin with disinfectant (on a small table).
Small cloth in basin.
Sandtimer.
Soap in soap dish.
Washbowls.

Procedure
1. Take a cloth from the solution.
2. Turn on faucet with cloth wet with disinfectant.
3. Take soap with same cloth.
4. Turn sandtimer over. This is contaminated so may be turned with the hand.

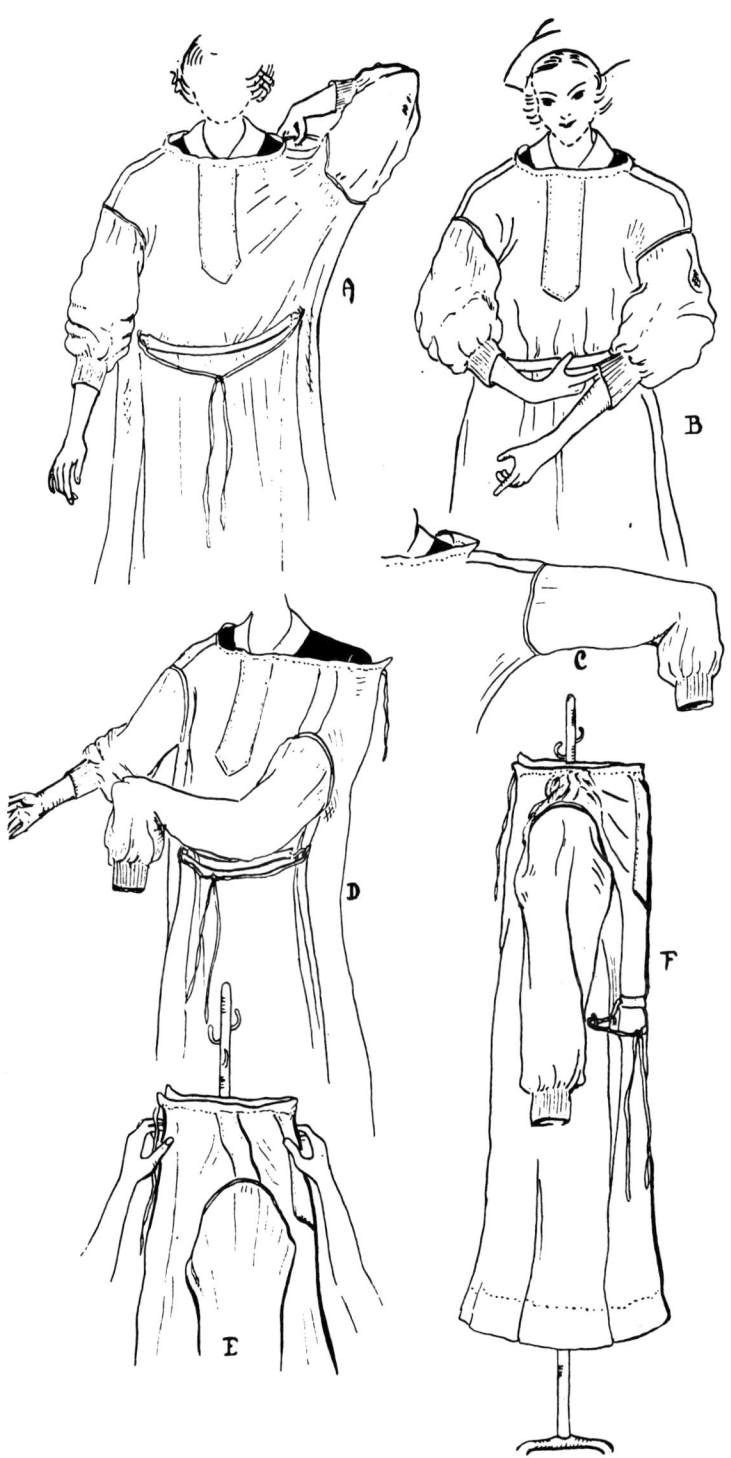

Sketches illustrating the technique of
removing the gown.

5. Scrub for 2 minutes. Use plenty of soap, rinse, resoap. Frequent soaping, rinsing, and resoaping is important in disinfecting. At the end of 2 minutes, rinse.
6. Dry hands well with paper toweling and turn off faucet with this paper.
7. Apply hand lotion.

In cases of measles, chicken pox, and smallpox, soak hands before drying for ½ minute in disinfectant, kept on shelf of table.

CARE OF HANDS IN THE UNIT: BEFORE REMOVING GOWN

This procedure is necessary to render hands clean before drawing them through inside gown.

Method no. 1, used in individual rooms:

Necessary articles in unit
Basin of disinfectant. In this method the hands are rinsed in the solution for about ½ minute. They are not dried.

Method no. 2, used in wards when there are several individual units:

Necessary articles
Clean washbowl.
Basin of disinfectant in which is placed a small cloth.
Soap in soap dish.

Procedure
1. When you are ready to remove gown and have pulled your sleeves up, go to washbowl, but do not touch it; you are contaminated, the washbowl is clean.
2. Take cloth from solution.
3. Turn on faucets.
4. Take bar of soap and scrub for 1 minute.
5. Your hands are now clean; turn off your faucets. Do not dry.
6. Remove gown.

WARD ROUTINE

Order of morning work
1. Consult kardex and patient's chart. Acquaint yourself with the treatment he is to receive. Go to your patient, greet him, observe and still further anticipate his needs.
2. Make a survey of the room to determine what is needed.
3. Get everything ready before becoming contaminated:
   a. Carry into room the necessary supplies, such as linen, soap, paper bag, cleaning cloth, solution of gargle, ice water, ice for ice collars, watch on towel, etc.
   b. Place hamper bag outside of door.
4. Be sure that mask is well over mouth and nose.
5. Put on isolation gown.

6. Assemble materials.
7. Give patient necessary care:
   a. Bedpan or urinal; have patient wash hands.
   b. Cleanse the mouth.
   c. Give bath.
   d. Give care to nails.
8. Make bed. Tuck in all bedclothes, including spread, on each side of bed to prevent clothing from slipping to floor and becoming contaminated. No linen, contaminated or clean, should touch the floor.
9. Place used linen in hamper bag outside the door.
10. Place towel over pillow; comb patient's hair; remove towel.
11. See that all utensils are clean and in place. See that your unit is scrupulously clean.
12. Pin paper bag to bed.
13. Before removing gown, see that materials to be taken from room are assembled and placed where you can take them after the gown is removed without contaminating your ward uniform.
14. Remove gown as taught. Hang on hook.
15. Empty hand solution basin, clean, and place in its brace empty.
16. Take with you from the room the soiled paper bag and utensils to be sterilized. Put the utensils in their respective places. Put trash in incinerator. Open incinerator with clean elbow.
17. Scrub in outer scrub room for 2 minutes.
18. Tie linen bag as taught, wheel it to linen chute, and drop it in chute.
19. Burn contents in incinerator.
20. While still clean, take broom and dustpan from closet. The handles are clean. Sweep your unit without becoming contaminated. Replace broom and dustpan, having burned in incinerator anything collected. (You may sweep all units at one time unless any individual one requires immediate attention.)
21. Make up a solution of disinfectant and pour into basin in unit without becoming contaminated.
22. Ask your patient if he is comfortable and if there is anything he wishes.

Serving of meals

Trays are prepared in the kitchen and carried to the patient's rooms. The aim of the nurse must be not to contaminate herself in any way. The tray is placed on the corner of the patient's table or on the edge of his bed and pushed into place by placing fingers against the inner, uncontaminated edge of the tray. The door is pushed open with the foot.

Collecting dinner trays

1. From the cart (stretcher) remove the padding.
2. Open sterilizer.
3. Remove cover of garbage can.
4. Place on cart a container for solid waste and one for liquid waste.
5. Remove trays from the patients' rooms and place on cart. To remove a tray: open the door with the elbow, place hand inside of the contaminated tray, pull toward you until part of the tray is over the edge of the bed portable so that you can grasp it with the other hand without touching anything but the tray. Then push the door open with the foot and place the tray on the cart. (When the nurse has carried the first tray, her hands are contaminated. Her aim must be to avoid touching anything except the tray in the patient's room.)
6. Scrape and stack dishes, putting solid and liquid waste in respective receptacles; food remnants are placed in the garbage can in the kitchen and liquids are poured into the hopper in the mop closet. *Nothing* contaminated is poured into the kitchen sink. The cart is contaminated.
7. Place dishes and trays in sterilizer in kitchen.
8. Scrub hands for 2 minutes.
9. Close door of sterilizer, turn on the steam, and allow the dishes to sterilize for 20 minutes.
10. Replace cover on garbage can.
11. Take a cleaning cloth and bar of soap, turn on faucet in scrub room, and thoroughly wash cart with soap and water. Do not rinse until hands have been scrubbed.
12. Scrub 2 minutes.
13. Rinse and dry cart. Replace pad. See that it is neatly covered with the sheet.
14. The maid will turn off the sterilizer and wash the dishes.

Passing medicines: a clean procedure

1. Assemble on tray the medications that are to be given to those of your patients who are able to take their own medicines.
2. Go to first patient's bedside.
3. Place medicine glass on bedside table without touching the table or any article on it.
4. Stand by the bed (do not let your uniform become contaminated) until the patient has taken the medication.
5. If he has no water on the bedside table, pour water from your tray pitcher into his empty medicine glass. Do not let the pitcher touch the glass or become contaminated in any other way.

6. Ask the patient to place his glass on the table. Leave it there. Do not touch it or return it to your tray.
7. Open the door with your foot. Leave the unit and go to the next patient, repeating the foregoing procedure.
8. When all medicines are passed to your group, put the tray in the medicine cabinet and begin to collect the glasses.

Note. — In giving medication to very ill patients, the nurse must put on the unit gown and assist the patient in taking the medicine. If giving of medication correlates in time with the morning and evening care, it may be given as any other treatment.

Collecting medicine glasses
1. Enter unit (when contaminated, open door with elbow).
2. Pick up medicine glass by top without touching anything else in the unit. If this is done correctly, you are contaminated, but the patient is not contaminated with any disease other than the one he has.
3. Carry this glass in one hand.
4. Go to next unit. Repeat procedure.
5. Wash medicine glasses in the utility room. *They must not be washed in the kitchen.*
6. Place in dishpan on stove. Scrub hands in utility room for 2 minutes.
7. Label the pan by pinning on the handle a red tag marked "contaminated," on which is written, "The inside of this pan is contaminated until this tag is removed."
8. Boil 20 minutes. Remove tag. Wash medicine glasses.

Watches
1. Necessary articles:
Watch.
Safety pin.
Towel.
2. Procedure:
   a. In taking T. P. R.'s during morning or evening care, before becoming contaminated, pin watch on a clean folded towel, but do not pin through bottom layer. It is placed on stand in unit without nurse becoming contaminated. When contaminated, the nurse can place hand under bottom of towel and pick up watch. When finished taking the unit pulses and respirations, place towel back on stand or other convenient place. Be sure it is out of patient's reach if patient is likely to reach for it. Watch is not removed until the hands are clean. Then remove watch and leave towel. This may be used in the unit later. The watch has been kept clean.

b. If watch should become contaminated, wash off with alcohol. Do this, when clean, by grasping watch with alcohol sponge. When this area is clean, take this part of watch in other hand and finish cleaning watch.

Routine duties of relief nurse, 7 p. m.–11 p. m.

1. Make rounds at least once every hour. Give special attention to those requiring it.
2. Carry out all treatments and medications when due between 7 p. m. and 11 p. m.
3. Pass nourishments.
4. Pass fresh water.
5. Take elevated temperatures and chart them.
6. Try to have all routine work done by 9 p. m. so that lights can be turned out.
7. Check and chart all medications and treatments.
8. Chart unusual condition of patients.
9. Charting is to be done in red from 7 p. m. to 7 a. m.
10. Make out temperature sheet and condition slips.
11. The relief nurse is responsible for carrying out and copying all new orders on order sheet of patient chart and for making out kardex and medicine cards. Copy all orders on order sheet in red from 7 p. m. to 7 a. m.
12. Check narcotics with night nurse at 11 p. m.
13. Make rounds with night nurse.
14. Report off duty to night supervisor in Annex Office.

Routine duties of night nurse, 11 p. m.–7 a. m.

1. While on duty, never leave your station uncovered. Call night supervisor for any assistance or relief.
2. Check narcotics with relief nurse at 11 p. m. and with dressing room nurse at 7 a. m. Report any missing narcotics to head nurse at once.
3. Make rounds with relief nurse and thereafter at least once every hour.
4. Copy orders written after 11 p. m. on order sheets and on kardex and make out medication cards. (Single orders are not copied on kardex or medication cards.)
5. Draw midnight lines on charts, date temperature sheets, and record intakes and diets.
6. Clean scrub room every night. Change solution in disinfectant basin.
7. Collect empty medicine bottles and put in drug basket.
8. Empty waste baskets and hamper bags.
9. Clean and scrub desks, chairs, and ink wells in hall, telephone booth, and office every night. Change pen points P. R. N.

10. Pass wash water and mouthwash to all patients every morning, starting in time to finish by 7 A. M.
11. Have report ready by 6 A. M.
12. Collect pitchers and mouthwash cups from all rooms every day and boil for 20 minutes in kitchen sterilizer. Boil drinking tubes and glasses in soda solution in dishpan. Do not forget to record amount taken from pitcher.
13. Collect urine specimens as per routine orders after midnight. Scarlet fever on Tuesday and Saturday mornings, all others on Wednesday A. M. Routine admission specimen on night of admission.
14. Report to the head nurse in writing all specimens not obtained. Try again the next night.
15. Rule the order book and date for 7 A. M.
16. See that the dressing room, kitchen, and scrub room are in order before reporting off duty. Remove all instruments from phenol and alcohol and put in their proper places.
17. Tidy rooms and wards. Straighten patients' beds; see that all bedding is straight and properly tucked in. It is not necessary to awaken infants for special A. M. care, but be sure that they are dry and properly covered at all times and that feedings are given regularly.
18. Report to head nurse in writing all broken, borrowed, or lost articles every morning before going off duty.

Cleaning and Care of Contaminated Articles

Methods of sterilization and cleaning contaminated articles
Note. — Whenever the material permits, articles to be sterilized should first be scrubbed with soap and water.

1. Boiling: 20 minutes unless otherwise specified.
   a. In a dish sterilizer: dishes, trays, enamel pitchers, kitchen utensils, white enamel cups. nursing bottles, etc.
   b. In dishpan: drinking tubes, medicine glasses.
   c. In instrument sterilizer: White enamel ware, such as kidney basins, soap dishes, dressing bowls, etc.
      Surgical instruments (not sharp).
      Speculi (first to be cleaned with applicators and washed), needles, syringes, etc.
      Rubber tubing, soft rubber catheters, rectal tubes, rubber gloves (time for each as previously taught).
      Metal toys.
2. By steam pressure in autoclave:
   a. Surgical supplies, rubber gloves, etc.
   b. Letters.

3. By scrubbing with soap and water:
   a. Large utensils of enamel ware, such as bathtubs, bedpans, wash basins.
   b. Stethoscope.
   c. Rubber sheets, hot-water bottles, icecaps, etc.
4. By placing in antiseptic solution:
   a. Sharp instruments such as scalpels, scissors, etc.
   b. Thermometers, wash with soap and water, place in antiseptic for 20 minutes.
   c. Intubation tubes.
5. By sunlight and fresh air for at least 6 hours:
   a. Leather goods such as restraint straps and cuffs, suitcases and patient's clothing, mattresses and pillow.
   b. Leather slippers.
   c. Light extension cords.
6. A volcanic ash and ammonium chloride:
   For furniture. (This is to prevent removal of paint and yet free the article from contamination.) Add ½ ounce of ammonium chloride to 2 gallons of water in which there is volcanic ash.

Sweeping

This is to be done when you are clean. No extra gown is necessary. Brooms and dustpans are found in the mop closet. The handles are kept clean. The bristles of the broom and the pan of dust are of course contaminated. When you have finished your morning cares and are clean, take a broom and dustpan. Go to your first unit and sweep. The broom handle is to touch nothing. Sweep sweepings into dustpan. Your hands and handle should still be clean. Go to your next unit. Proceed as above. When finished, burn sweepings in incinerator. Return broom and pan to mop closet.

Lights

Electric lights are to be turned off and on with clean paper.

Radiators

Radiators are to be turned off and on with clean paper.

Windows

Windows are to be opened and closed with clean paper.

Incinerator

The door of the incinerator and the walls surrounding it must be kept clean. When your hands are contaminated, open the incinerator with your clean elbow. Do not overload the incinerator. The door must be kept closed. As soon as you are clean, burn the contents. If it is necessary to use the poker, take handle with a piece of clean paper.

Cleaning washbowls

When clean, scrub everything above bowl with a clean cloth and soap. Start with soap dish, then clean faucet, etc. Rinse this part well. Now do bowl. Start at upper edge. The inside is done last. Clean from top to bottom, the outlet being the last part to be scrubbed. The bowl is clean, the nurse's hands contaminated. Discard cloth in hamper bag. Scrub hands 2 minutes.

Note. — Although at the end of this procedure the bowl is clean, it must always be considered contaminated because it is constantly receiving contaminated washings. Never touch the bowl inside. The nurse should come in contact with it only when cleaning it.

Care of linen: hamper bags

Soiled linen is placed in hamper bags. Plain hamper bags are for sheets, pillowslips, towels, etc. Striped bags are for the dark clothes — bathrobes, blankets, stockings, etc. The hamper bag hangs on a hamper stand, the top edge pulled out and over the rim. Be sure there are no holes in the hamper bags. Hamper bags are to be two-thirds full only. Each nurse is to tie up her own hamper bag when it has reached the two-thirds mark. Do not leave this to be done by someone else. It is part of your duty.

To tie hamper bag

1. When ready to tie up hamper bag, loosen outer edge and let bag drop into center of hamper ring. It will rest on the metal triangle. It must not touch the floor. Holding the string in one hand, from the outside gather the top of the bag together. See that the edges of the opening are in proximity. Roll side opening inward. Wrap hamper drawstring around top. Secure it.
2. Pin a red "contaminated" tag on upper hem of bag, going through outer part of hem only.
3. Wheel the bag to the linen chute. Drop the bag down the chute. (The orderly will take the bag to the laundry, where the contents are rendered noncontaminated by washing.)
4. Return hamper stand to utility room and place a clean bag on the hamper stand.

Cleaning specimen containers

1. Spinal fluid specimens:
   a. In taking spinal fluid, the test tubes for specimens invariably become contaminated. When they have been collected, place them in an enamel container; this can be disinfected and need not be destroyed. (Before beginning the procedure, place a red "contaminated" tag under the container.)

b. Scrub hands for 2 minutes.

c. When hands are clean, grasp the tube with an alcohol sponge and cleanse part of it. In the other hand take this clean part and continue to clean the entire tube, omitting only the cotton stopper.

d. When alcohol has dried, flame cotton stopper and edge of tube. (If you do not wait until alcohol is dry, the flame will travel down the tube and burn your hands.)

e. Place tubes in pasteboard container, sent to laboratory with the laboratory request sheet.

2. Urine specimens:

a. In collecting urine specimens, take a bottle without cork into the unit. Consider it contaminated. Collect specimen. When clean, cleanse as above with alcohol sponge, cleaning top edge without letting alcohol enter specimen.

b. Take out of unit and place a clean cork in bottle. If it is a catheterized specimen and you have used the cotton pledget as a cork, still clean as above. Remove cotton pledget with the alcohol sponge, discard. Replace with a sterile stopper from the clean sterile dressing can.

Flashlights and otoscopes

Because these instruments have batteries within them, they must not be placed in a basin of disinfectant to clean. No moisture should reach the batteries.

1. Flashlight:

a. Wrap in paper towel and hand to doctor. When he has finished using it, he unwraps it as one would sterile goods and the nurse takes the clean flashlight. Should it become contaminated, clean with an alcohol sponge.

2. Otoscope:

a. Wrap in paper towel. The doctor tries to contaminate nothing but the speculum. When the examination is completed, the doctor removes the speculum, places it on the table and unwraps otoscope, and the nurse takes it. When the doctor goes to scrub, he takes with him the speculum, placing it in the washbowl. (It is later scrubbed with soap and water, placed in alcohol for 10 minutes, dried, and placed in otoscope box.)

b. If doctor needs the nurse's assistance during the procedure, he takes with him when he leaves the unit the wrapped otoscope and asks a clean nurse outside the unit to take it. If any part should become contaminated, clean with an alcohol sponge.

Mail

1. "Letters that are to go through the sterilizer before being mailed shall be placed in a plain envelope addressed in pencil. When letter is returned to the station, sterilized, the nurse there on duty shall place each envelope into a fresh envelope bearing the hospital name in the upper left hand corner, she herself addressing this new envelope."
2. When stamps are sent to the station, see that they are kept clean. This will necessitate opening packages before patients, under their observation, having first explained the reason and secured permission. The stamps are filed in a box for the purpose. Each patient's stamps are placed in a small envelope on which is written the patient's name. After addressing envelope, put on stamp. If the patient has no stamps, send the letter to the business office to be stamped.
3. Suggest to your patients that unless they wish to write letters of a very personal nature, they may have sent in to them some one-cent, plain postcards. These sterilize better. No extra stamps are necessary. Pencil should be used.
4. Each evening before 7 P. M. a nurse collects letters. Take a clean paper bag and make on it an outward cuff. Go to the bedside of the patients who can write letters and have them drop letters into the bag without contaminating the outside. Close the bag by turning up the cuff. Label with letter of station, date, and "Letters to be sterilized." Take to Sterile Supply Room. The package will be returned to the station the following morning. Then proceed as above.

Plants

A plant sent in usually lasts longer than the patient's isolation period. He may enjoy taking it home with him. Therefore keep the plant clean. It may be placed on a clean table. Label this table "clean" so no one will contaminate it. In a room have it in a corner not frequently passed. In a ward it may remain in the clean area. Water it when you are clean.

Visitors

1. No visiting is to be permitted in the Contagious Department except in the case of critically ill patients or where the professional staff feels that visits from the family or other individuals may have a definite therapeutic value in bringing about the recovery of the patient.
2. No visitors are to be admitted to the Contagious Department to see critically ill patients other than as set forth in the following schedule:
   a. Visiting shall be limited to 2 individuals on any one day.

b. If the father and mother are living only they shall be allowed to see the patient.

c. One other member of the family may be permitted as a substitute if either one of the parents is deceased.

d. If both father and mother are deceased or if father and mother are too far distant to visit patient, then a substitute visitor may be permitted in lieu of either of absent parents.

e. If the patient is a married adult, the husband or wife and one other relative, preferably the father or mother, may be permitted to see the patient once daily.

3. The visiting period is to be limited, preferably to 5 minutes, and in no instance is to exceed 10 minutes.

4. No visitors are to be permitted to enter the patient's room, but they may be permitted to see the patient through the window provided for that purpose or to converse with the patient from the doorway.

5. Visitors need not be gowned or capped where visiting is conducted in this manner.

6. Any visitor who enters a patient's room is to be held under arrest and not permitted to leave the Contagious Unit until he or she has conformed to all regulations required for a patient who is being discharged from this department, including antiseptic bath and a complete change of fresh clothing, which must be brought in, and a sterilization of all clothing worn at the time the patient's room was entered.

Draping wheeled stretcher (for taking patients to X-ray, etc.)

The stretcher is first draped in the usual manner, having on it a rubber pad covered with a sheet. A second sheet is placed on the stretcher lengthwise, single thickness. There must be no holes in the sheet. Fold the sides under the sheet itself. Have enough of the folded edge hanging over the sides of stretcher to protect them from contamination. These sides are later pulled out and up over the patient, making an externally clean unit.

Disinfection of stools and urine of typhoid and dysentery patients

1. Cover mass in bedpan with one cupful of chloride of lime. Use a sputum cup for this purpose.

2. Add enough hot water to cover the mass.

3. Mix contents well, using a spatula.

4. Empty contents of bedpan into enamel container for the purpose. If the contents are well mixed, they will leave the pan readily, leaving it grossly clean.

5. Without washing, boil bedpan for 20 minutes.

6. The contents of several bedpans may be placed in the container. One container receives them from 7 A. M. to 7 P. M., another from 7 P. M. to 7 A. M. The day container is emptied

at 9 P. M. and the night container at 9 A. M. Two hours is allowed for disinfection of last stool put in container.

7. Containers are thoroughly washed in soap and water and aired (sunned if possible) until next time used.

Note. — If no container is available, proceed through step 3. Cover with bedpan cover and allow bedpan to stand for 2 hours. Empty contents and wash bedpan. It may remain in patient's unit.

Disinfection of food from typhoid patients
Soiled food:
  Wrap in paper all soiled food remaining on patient's tray and burn in incinerator.
Liquid food:
  Empty liquid food into bedpan and care for as directed in procedure for "Disinfection of stools and urine."

Terminal disinfection of a unit
1. Necessary articles (clean) :
  Mattress cover. (There must be no holes in it.)
  12 safety pins.
  Cloth.
  Foot tub with 8 quarts warm water. Kidney basin which has a disinfectant in it.
  Cleaning cloth.
  1 cupful wall-washing powder.
  ½ oz. powdered ammonium chloride.
  Leave these articles outside unit until ready to use them.
2. Procedure:
  a. Put all articles on one end of cart. Make up in tub a washing solution of water, ammonium chloride, and wall-washing powder. Cover rest of cart with mattress cover and place outside of door of room that is to be scrubbed. Wheel hamper to door (in corridor).
  b. Enter the room and put on the gown (contaminated) that is hanging on the hook.
  c. Strip linen off bed and place in hamper bag.
  d. Fold mattress with pillows inside and put on cart in corridor. See that ends of mattress are folded under. Taking hold of inside of mattress cover, pull ends up and over mattress. Do not pin now.
  e. Spread rubber sheet on bed.
  f. Sort all articles in room. Leave nothing on bedside table.
  g. Remove contaminated gown.
  h. Place in dish sterilizer all dishes, mouth cups, pitchers, drinking tubes, etc.

i. Place in large sterilizer emesis basins, soap dish, tub, basins, etc. Be sure they are washed first.

j. Put trash in incinerator, opening it with clean elbow.

k. Scrub hands for 2 minutes.

l. Pin mattress cover. When pins are put into cover, they come in contact with inside of cover, which has been against mattress and is therefore contaminated. As this pin is pushed through on the outside again, before pinning wash point with the cloth wet in disinfectant. Brace pin point with this cloth and close it. Your fingers should not touch the part of pin going through cover. Pin on this covered mattress a red "contaminated" sign. Take mattress to corridor by elevators and leave on one of vacant beds. Discard cloth in laundry. Leave cart in proper place.

m. From foot tub in which is the cleaning solution take cleaning cloth, enter unit, and scrub top of bedside table. On the table place the clean foot tub. Finish cleaning bedside table. Touch nothing until you have first cleaned it. Be sure your uniform does not touch the furniture as you clean. If you contaminate your uniform, you may recontaminate the already cleaned furniture.

n. Scrub upper side of rubber sheet. Fold once and scrub the now upper half.

o. Scrub uncovered half of bed. Turn clean side of rubber sheet over onto clean part of bed. Finish scrubbing rubber sheet. Let it remain on the spring of bed while you continue to scrub room.

p. Finish scrubbing bed.

q. Scrub all furniture. Finish by scrubbing window sill and handles, shelf, fixtures, toilet, etc.

r. Invert bedside table and chairs and place on bed. Be sure the part touching floor does not come in contact with bed. Scrub feet of tables and chair. Leave bed, with all equipment on it, in middle of room.

s. Remove scrubbing equipment. Boil foot tub. Discard cloth in hamper bag. Scrub hands for 2 minutes. Turn card on door to vertical position. Take rubber sheet to roof for sunning and airing. Tie up laundry bag, label with red tag, place in chute.

t. The windows, walls, and floors are washed by the orderly. If the room is not to be used for the next twenty-four hours, but may be aired during this time, the windows and walls need not be washed.

u. When all cleaning and airing is completed, remove cards on door and place in their stead a card marked "Vacant and Disinfected." Make up room for a new patient.

Note. — Until the nurse goes in to clean the room, the cards naming the patient and the disease remain horizontally on the door. When the furniture has been scrubbed, but not the walls, the cards are placed in the vertical position. When the walls and the entire room are clean, place the "Vacant and Disinfected" sign on the door.

Care of dead in an isolated unit

1. Make preparations for giving the discharge bath in bed.
2. In addition, have tags and bandage as prescribed in procedure "Care of the Dead." Also have wheeled cart ready. In addition to the usual cover place on it a large sheet, draped as taught for isolated cases, and over this the morgue sheet. Have 6 safety pins on the cart. Leave cart just outside door in the corridor.
3. Give bath as directed in "Terminal Bed Bath," washing the hair with 70 per cent alcohol, instead of soap and water, also observing directions as in procedure "Care of the Dead." When both have been given, proceed as directed in 10, 11, and 12 under procedure "Care of the Dead." Place a clean towel over patient.
4. Wheel cart into room. Keep it clean.
5. Place patient on cart. Remove towel. Wrap in the morgue sheet as directed in "Care of the Dead."
6. A clean nurse, according to technique, covers the body with the second sheet.
7. The body is to be taken to the morgue in basement of the contagion building. When you are ready to leave the floor, call the Annex Office and request that door to morgue be opened for you. Take with you a card 3x½ inches with the patient's name on it. With this label door on icebox. In placing patient in icebox, both sheets are left around patient. When body has been taken care of, lock door, return keys to Annex Office, and return cart to station.

Assisting with Treatments and Examinations

Taking cultures

1. Fill out regulation culture slip for each patient to have cultures taken. Take the same number of culture tubes, sets of applicators, and elastic bands. The tubes are sterile inside. The applicators also are sterile, all but the ends being sealed in a small envelope.
2. If the patient is cooperative, both doctor and nurse remain clean, the nurse holding the culture tube while the doctor takes culture from nose with one applicator and from throat with the other. If the applicators are placed in the tube with-

out touching the edge, the cotton stopper is replaced and no disinfecting of tube is necessary. (If the tube becomes contaminated, it is treated as is a spinal fluid specimen.) Wrap the correct slip around the tube. Secure with elastic band.

3. Go to next patient.
4. If it is necessary to hold the patient while the cultures are being taken, the doctor can hold the slips and stopper and tubes in one hand and take cultures with the other. The nurse holds the patient. She then scrubs for 2 minutes and returns to assist with other cultures.
5. The cultures must be in the Annex Office before 8 A. M. and 7 P. M.

Technique for assisting laboratory technicians (blood counts)

1. Equipment:
Alcohol sponge.
Large sheet of paper (newspaper) or hand towel.
Laboratory request blank filled in, ready for the laboratory.
2. Procedure:
The nurse accompanies the doctor or technician, taking with her the large sheet of paper and a sponge wet with alcohol.
   a. Place sheet of paper (or towel) on bedside table and instruct doctor or technician to place the paper on this tray. Letter it, "In no way touch any contaminated article." (The table should be completely covered and part of the paper should hang over the front. In this way the tubing with the pipette, as it swings while being held between the technician's teeth, will not swing against the uncovered table and become contaminated.)
   b. Ask the patient to extend the nearer hand. (Wash the hand with the alcohol sponge and instruct patient not to let the hand become contaminated.)
   c. The technician now works from the clean tray to the cleaned hand. If he touches only the tray and this hand, he need not wear a gown and need not scrub. (Since he shakes the white count tube by holding open ends of tube between his fingers, it would be well for him to wash his fingers on the outside of the alcohol sponge.) The slide and pipette are placed on the laboratory sheet, which the nurse holds in one hand. Later she fastens these to the laboratory sheet with labels. Unless the nurse has had to hold an uncooperative patient, she need not become contaminated during the procedure.
   d. Open the door with the foot. Take clean articles only with you.

Smears:
1. With a gummed label, fasten slide to a laboratory sheet. A clean nurse holds this for the doctor while he makes the smear. The doctor touches nothing but the upper surface of the slide. When the slide is dry, send to laboratory. A clean nurse holds a clean slide for the doctor. When smear has been made, let it dry. At each end, on side of smear, place a toothpick. Place a clean slide over the smear. The toothpicks will keep it from touching smear. Keep slide in place with an elastic band at each end. Wrap in clean paper. Send slide to laboratory.

Assisting doctor in taking blood pressure
1. Necessary articles:
2 hand towels (for 1 may be substituted a full sheet of newspaper).
Alcohol sponge.
Patient's gown (large size). A cuff of about 2 inches should be made on sleeve that would ordinarily go on arm nearer you.
Stethoscope.
Sphygmomanometer.
2. Procedure:
One nurse, clean, can do this, if patient is able to cooperate. If not, two nurses, one contaminated, one clean, are needed.
a. Without becoming contaminated, place a clean towel (or the newspaper) on bedside table. Be sure that side of table toward bed is covered. On this place the sphygmomanometer.
b. Slip cuffed sleeve of gown over arm near you and let rest of gown drape bed.
c. With the alcohol cloth cleanse the arm around the entire circumference for an area extending at least 3 inches above and below elbow.
d. Turn down cuff of gown, being careful not to touch contaminated edge. This makes a clean margin on the gown. It should come down well over disinfected area, leaving free the inner disinfected surface of elbow.
e. Cover hand and lower arm with clean towel. (This may be omitted if you feel you can avoid touching contaminated hand. One usually can when the patient is cooperative.)
f. Wrap arm band of sphygmomanometer over sleeve. It must not become contaminated.
g. The doctor now takes the blood pressure. He needs no gown. His stethoscope also remains clean because of disinfecting of the arm.

h. Remove sphygmomanometer while clean.
i. Re-enter unit. Remove articles used for draping. Make patient comfortable.
j. Scrub hands for 2 minutes.

Assisting X-ray technician in taking X-ray at bedside
1. Necessary articles:
Pillowslip without holes.
X-ray equipment.
2. Procedure:
   a. Before entering unit, explain to technician that the machine must be kept clean and that, if possible, the cord should be kept off the floor.
   b. Let the technician place the casette in the pillowslip.
   c. Enter unit and put on isolation gown.
   d. Take the covered casette from the technician and place it under patient as the technician directs you.
   e. When X-ray is taken, uncover the plate by making an outward cuff on the pillowship. The technician takes the plate without becoming contaminated.
   f. Make patient comfortable. Remove gown. Scrub for 2 minutes.
   g. If the cord to the machine has touched the floor, it must be cleansed with a cloth of alcohol. A clean person grasps the cord with the cloth. When one section is clean, this may be taken with the clean hand and the cloth is then drawn through the alcohol cloth.
   h. In the event that moisture comes in contact with the pillowslip on the casette, the entire outside of the plate must be washed with alcohol.

Assisting X-ray technician in taking X-ray in the X-ray department
The patient is on the stretcher completely wrapped in a clean sheet. After the nurse has turned back the sheet and has carefully removed from the part to be X-rayed clothing and anything else that would influence the result of the X-ray, the technician places the casette under the clean sheet. (The nurse is contaminated and so must not touch the casette.) The X-ray is taken. The technician removes the casette. The nurse makes the patient comfortable, covers patient again by grasping inner contaminated side of sheet, washes her hands in soap and water for 2 minutes. The patient is then taken back to the station.
Note.—If casette becomes contaminated in any way, wash off with alcohol.

Assisting doctors with dressing trays, hypodermoclysis, etc.
There must always be one clean nurse to serve the doctor. If the

patient is cooperative, this nurse will be the only one needed. If the patient is uncooperative, a second nurse should put on a gown and assist.

1. Set up tray, prepare solutions, etc., in the clean dressing room. (If tests such as the Dick, Schick, etc., are to be done, have the doctor fill the syringes while he is clean.) Nothing contaminated is to go on the tray.

2. On bedside table place a clean towel or newspaper, keeping upper side clean. On this place the clean, sterile tray. Have with you also, clean, the jar of handling forceps. Either on one corner of the unsterile part of tray or on a clean part of table place a clean emesis basin having under it a red "contaminated" sign.

3. Serve the doctor anything he wishes from the tray. He should not help himself. He discards articles used in the basin, coming in contact with inside only.

4. When the procedure is completed, the tray should be clean. Take it from the unit, care for it as you would on any other service.

5. Take contaminated articles from room. Scrub, boil if they permit of boiling.

   Note.—In the event that you are alone in the ward, as during relief, for instance, take the emesis basin by the clean outside. Place it by the clean tray. Keep the red tag under it so no one will touch it. Next time you become contaminated, scrub these articles and boil them if they can be boiled. If the articles must be boiled immediately, clean and boil them.

6. Scrub hands for 2 minutes.

Weighing an isolated baby

1. The scales are to remain clean.

2. A clean nurse weighs the sheet to be used around the contaminated baby. Having weighed it, she opens the sheet and holds it in her arms, ready to receive the child when the contaminated nurse places the child in her arms. The sheet is wrapped around the child. All of it must be included in the weighing. The clean nurse weighs the child, the scales remain clean. The child and sheet are returned to the nurse in the unit. (Since the scales are clean and only a clean sheet comes in contact with them, the sheet may be used in the unit.)

3. Subtract weight of sheet from combined weight of sheet and baby. Record the difference.

How a patient may sign a document without contaminating it

1. Necessary articles:
   Chart back.

Hand towel.

Pen, the handle of which is wrapped in paper.

2. Procedure
   a. Put document on chart back.
   b. Cover chart back and document with a towel, having upper edge even with line of signature and lower edge well below lower edge of chart back. (The patient's arm will not in that case contaminate the chart back as he writes.) Hand it to patient, instructing him not to touch document. The nurse holds the side that patient is not holding.
   c. Dip pen in ink and hand to patient, instructing him to touch only the paper.
   d. When the document has been signed, ask the patient to hold on to the towel and take out from the top the chart back and document. The patient holds the pen so that the nurse can take the clean upper part and remove it clean from the paper.
   e. The patient may put the towel on his side table and the paper from the pen in his paper bag.
   f. The nurse returns the chart back to the chart rack and places the document in its proper place.

Terminal Baths

Purpose
1. To prepare a patient who has had a contagious disease and his surroundings so that both she and her surroundings will be free from lingering infection after she is released from isolation.

THE TUB BATH

General instructions
1. If the patient is strong enough, she may have a tub or shower bath; if unable to be out of bed, a bed bath is given.

Necessary articles
   In the bathroom:
   Face towel.
   2 bath towels, 1 to dry patient and 1 to wrap around hair when leaving room.
   Washcloth.
   Bar of soap.
   Cup containing liquid soap for hair.
   Large pitcher of warm water for rinsing hair.
   Mattress pad.
   Pair slippers.

Pair pajamas.
Bathrobe.
Basin with cleaning cloth and disinfectant.
Large sheet.
In clean room to which patient is taken after bath:
Comb.
Patient's own clean clothing.
Mouthwash and emesis basin.

Preparation of equipment

1. Prepare clean bathroom, close window and door; have temperature not lower than 80° F. and free from drafts.
2. Fill tub half full of water at about 105° F.
3. Place washcloth on edge of tub with soap on it.
4. Have pitcher and cup with liquid soap on wide edge of tub.
5. Clothes, towels, etc., may be placed on chair.
6. Basin with disinfectant and cloth is placed on window ledge.

Preparation of patient

1. The nurse, in her clean uniform, takes a large clean sheet, folded once, and goes to the patient's unit. The patient is to be wrapped in this clean sheet before leaving the room to go to the bathroom. The nurse remains clean.
2. Explain to the patient what you wish to do.
3. If the patient is an adult:
   a. Have her put slippers on and remove all clothing but her gown.
   b. Have her stand away from the bed, back to the nurse, hands close to her sides.
   c. Wrap sheet around patient without contaminating yourself. Outside of sheet must be kept clean.
   d. Holding sheet and supporting patient, take patient to bathroom.
4. If the patient is a very young child, 2 nurses will be needed:
   a. The assistant (the clean nurse) holds across her arms the large sheet folded once.
   b. The nurse who is to bathe the child undresses him and places him in the sheet.
   c. She grasps the inner side of the sheet at the edge and covers the child.
   d. The clean nurse carries the child to the tub and puts him directly into it, the sheet still around him. The lower edge of the sheet becomes wet and contaminated. The child sits in the tub; if necessary, the nurse whose hands are contaminated to him may assist the child. Lift the sheet over the dry end and remove over faucet end of tub, drop to

floor. If this method is used, the tub must be cleaned where water from the sheet has dripped; for this use the cloth from the disinfectant solution, returning it to the solution. The nurse who is contaminated to the patient continues with the procedure, soaping her hands well before beginning the bath.

e. The clean nurse takes the child to the bathroom; the contaminated nurse, from inside the sheet, opens the sheet and lifts the child out and into the tub. If the child touches the edge of tub or wall, wash contaminated area with the cloth from the disinfectant solution.

Procedure

1. Explain what is to be kept clean in the room; gain patient's confidence and cooperation.
2. Supporting her and with sheet still around her, ask her to step out of slippers and stand on them.
3. Drop sheet to floor without letting it touch tub or walls.
4. Assist patient in stepping into tub. Her gown should not touch edge of tub. She may support herself on window ledge above faucet. If tub becomes contaminated, clean with disinfectant cloth.
5. While standing in tub have her remove gown and drop it on top of sheet without touching anything clean. Assist her to sit down in tub.
6. Wet her hair, apply soap and make a good suds; leave suds on hair, gathering it up on top of her head, and let it remain soaped until bath is finished.
7. Finish bathing patient or supervise her in bathing herself.
8. Rinse hair with water from pitcher.
9. Wring out washcloth and drop on contaminated linen. Place soap on edge of tub, open drain.
10. Have patient stand up in tub; let her dry herself while the nurse dries her back and places the doubled mattress pad on the floor.
11. Clothe patient, keeping clothing from touching floor.
12. Place second bath towel around patient's hair.
13. Take to clean room to await discharge.

After-care of patient

1. Help her dry her hair and make comfortable.
2. Instruct her about keeping free from contamination.

After-care of equipment

1. Leave bathroom door open.
2. Take soap in left hand and the cloth from the disinfectant solution in the right hand; soap cloth well.

    a. Clean window if patient touched it.
    b. Wash faucets.
    c. Wash around entire circumference. Continue overlapping each layer around tub all down sides.
    d. When bottom is reached, start at head of tub and wash toward outlet.
    e. Clean outlet last.
    f. Place soap on edge of tub; put cloth with soilèd linen.
    g. Your hands are now considered contaminated.
3. Place linen in linen bag in service room.
4. Burn slippers in incinerator.
5. Boil pitcher in kitchen sterilizer.
6. While tub is soaping for 2 minutes, scrub hands.
7. Rinse tub.

THE SHOWER BATH

General instructions
1. The shower is used when the patient is strong enough to take her own bath.
2. It may be used for patients who can take their own bath if they can be seated; in that case provide a stool.

Necessary articles
Same as tub bath.
Omit pitcher for rinsing hair.
Add stool, when needed.

Preparation of equipment
Omit filling tub with water.

Preparation of patient
Same as steps 1, 2, 3 in "The Tub Bath."

Procedure
1–3. As in "The Tub Bath."
4. Let patient drop gown on top of sheet.
5. Have patient step under shower so as to get hair and entire body wet.
6. Soap hair and body thoroughly and completely.
7. Rinse well.
8. Place folded mattress pad on floor and have patient step onto this to dry herself.
9. Clothe and place second bath towel around hair.
10. Take to room to await discharge.

After-care of patient
1. Help her dry her hair and make comfortable.
2. Instruct her about keeping free from contamination.

After-care of equipment
 1. Clean walls of shower as sides of bath tub were cleaned.
 2. When walls are finished, empty basin of disinfectant over the floor.

INFANT'S BATH

General instructions
 1. The nurse puts on a clean isolation gown, but remains clean during the procedure. The gown is merely for protection should the infant splash water.
 2. The hands of the nurse will be as clean as the infant when the bath is finished.

Necessary articles
 2 clean bedside tables.
 Bathtub.
 Washcloth.
 Soap in soap dish.
 Mattress pad.
 Bath towel.
 Clean clothing.
 Clean isolation gown.

Preparation of equipment
 1. Collect equipment, fill tub one-third full with water 105°.
 2. On one clean stand place the tub of water, soap in dish, and washcloth.
 3. On second stand place the mattress pad, opened to cover top of stand. On this place the bath towel.
 4. Place the infant's clean clothing on the shelf of the second stand.

Preparation of patient.
 1. Put on clean isolation gown.
 2. Undress infant and place him in the water, being careful that only the hands are contaminated.

Procedure
 1. Give a complete bath; except for her hands the nurse remains clean.
 2. Lift infant out of tub, place on towel on second stand, and wrap him up for a minute in the towel and pad so he will remain warm.
 3. Dry well and clothe.

After-care of patient
 1. Take to clean unit to await discharge.

After-care of equipment
 1. Equipment may be cleaned when unit is cleared.

2. Remove gown.
3. Scrub hands for 2 minutes.

DISCHARGE BATH IN BED

General instructions
1. Two nurses are needed for this procedure — one in the gown contaminated to the patient and one in a clean isolation gown.
2. The clean nurse must remain clean during the entire procedure. Whenever the clean nurse needs assistance, the contaminated nurse either helps with the contaminated part, or the clean nurse cleans the contaminated nurse's hands so she can assist with the clean parts of the procedure. Often a paralyzed poliomyelitis patient cannot be cared for without assistance from both nurses.
3. If this bath is given to a deceased patient, a basin of alcohol is needed. The hair is washed with alcohol and after soaping and rinsing each part, it is sponged with alcohol. Then proceed as in "Care of the Dead."

Necessary articles
Foot tub with warm water.
Cupful of liquid soap.
Large pitcher of warm water.
Bar of soap in soap dish.
2 washcloths.
Face towel.
3 bath towels.
Kelly pad.
Gown (patient's).
Blanket.
Mattress pad.
2 large sheets. Fold each sheet once, hem to hem, roll in one side of sheet.
Isolation gown (clean).

Preparation of equipment — by clean nurse
1. Collect all necessary articles and carry to patient's bed.
2. Place articles on a clean table far enough from patient's bed so that they will not become contaminated.

Preparation of patient — by contaminated nurse
1. Move bed to center of room.
2. Remove upper bedclothes, replacing with a bath blanket.
3. Remove patient's gown.
4. Have patient lie diagonally across bed, pillow under shoulders ready for shampoo. This shampoo is always given at the side

of the bed because there is less danger of the nurse contaminating herself.

5. Place patient's foot tub on chair at side and head of bed.

Procedure — by the clean nurse with contaminated nurse assisting

1. Shampoo the hair.
   a. Place Kelly pad under patient's head without contaminating yourself.
   b. From pitcher pour water over patient's hair.
   c. Pour liquid soap on hair and soap hair thoroughly, guiding Kelly pad so that it does not fall from bed; have patient raise head. Wash back of neck. Wash the part of Kelly pad under neck and head of patient.
   d. While hair is soaping, wash patient's face and anterior part of neck.
   e. Rinse hair well. Let Kelly pad drop into foot tub. Contaminated nurse will remove chair with tub and pad.
   f. Place folded mattress pad under patient's head after he has moved back to center of bed. Have it wide enough to come down to shoulders. Wrap bath towel around head. Be sure it does not touch contaminated head of bed.
2. Have contaminated nurse uncover the arm nearest you. With washcloth in right hand, wash wrist of arm near you. With left hand grasp clean wrist and continue to wash hand and arm of patient. Dry. Keep arm, washcloth, towel, and yourself away from contaminated bed. Place clean arm on pad under head.
3. Have contaminated nurse uncover patient to hips. Wash patient from neck to hips, washing and drying a small part at a time.
4. Have assistant uncover part of thigh nearest you. Wash.
5. As contaminated nurse draws blanket down to knees, place small towel over pubes. (The top edge and side nearest you are clean and this is very important later.) With clean hand patient holds this towel in place as she turns.
6. Turn patient on side so face is away from you. (The contaminated nurse watches patient so that no part that is already clean becomes contaminated.) Wash back from neck to knees. Rinse. Dry. Be careful that towel does not touch bed. Be sure that you in no way become contaminated.
7. Place one sheet on bed so roll is at patient's back and so that it overlaps about 6 inches of mattress pad. It is large enough to reach almost to knees.
8. Have patient turn on back. Put clean arm into sleeve of gown and cover patient halfway across chest and to waistline.

9. Take (as with first arm) the arm farthest from you. Wash. Dry.
10. Have patient turn toward you. (She merely rolls over. Patients seem to have tendency, unless warned, so to shift the buttocks that clean side rests on contaminated bed. This will not happen if she merely rolls over onto side.) She holds towel over pubes with hand nearest you. Since the edge of towel near you is clean, it cannot contaminate clean sheet now on bed.
11. Wash rest of patient's back to knees. Dry.
12. From clean side of roll, unroll sheet so that it covers farthest side of bed.
13. Have patient turn on back.
14. Put gown on other arm; upper part of body should now be covered to waistline. Bed is clean from top to halfway between hips and knees, except pubic region. Patient's back from neck to knees is clean.
15. Fanfold blanket and place across patient's chest. Continue to cover patient as bath is given.
16. Place towel on patient's chest so that it will be ready for patient to use. Hand patient a well-soaped washcloth. Have it wrung out well. Instruct her to lift towel from pubes so that it does not drag across her or the bed and drop it to floor. Have her finish her bath. (You may have to rinse cloth for her.) She dries with towel on chest, having been instructed not to let it go beyond clean area. She brings gown down to a line halfway between knees and hips, since lower part of bed is clean to this distance only.
17. With second washcloth, proceed with bath.
18. Have contaminated nurse uncover leg near you. Wash this leg and foot, using method as for arm.
19. Wash one hand of contaminated nurse and have her hold patient's leg from bed while you get second sheet.
20. Place sheet on bed with upper part overlapping at least 6 inches of first sheet, roll coming to center of bed. Place leg on sheet. Cover with bath towel until you need it.
21. Have nurse with her contaminated hand remove contaminated blanket from other leg. Wash other leg and foot as the first. Unroll sheet so that it covers other half of bed. Place patient's leg on bed.
22. Cover legs with bath blanket.
23. Dry patient's hair and comb it.

RECORD OF PROFICIENCY IN NURSING PRACTICE

Name	Service	Day
Class	Ward	Night
Hospital	From	To

I. Professional Aptitudes and Skills:

A. Consider the accuracy with which the student carries out practical nursing procedures.

Procedures usually carried out as taught.   Carries out procedures as taught.   Very careless and negligent of detail.

B. Consider the ability with which the student makes a plan for carrying out the duties assigned her.

Cannot arrange tasks without aid.   Fair organization — occasionally needs assistance to make good plan.   Makes workable plan.

C. Consider ability to adjust to ward situations.

Judgment shown in reacting to ward situations is poor.   Usually meets situations adequately.   Always makes satisfactory adjustment.

D. Consider tact in dealing with doctors, associates, and patients.

Antagonizes doctors, patients, or associates.*   Usually tactful.   Extremely tactful. Wins confidence of associates, patients, and doctors.

E. Consider student's powers of observation.

Fails to note details or symptoms.   Usually observes details or symptoms.   Displays keen powers of observation.

F. Consider the trustworthiness of the student.

Cannot be depended on.   Usually trustworthy.   Always trustworthy.

G. Consider the interest shown in seizing opportunities to learn.

Indifferent to opportunity of adding to knowledge or skill.   Moderately eager to improve.   Always eager to learn.

H. Consider the development of student while in this department.

Showed little improvement.   Fair amount of progress.   Marked development.

I. Consider the student's loyalty to school policies.

Faultfinding, insincere.*   Usually loyal.   Always loyal and enthusiastic.

J. Consider quality of written work—reports, charts, etc.; neatness, accuracy, completeness.

Written work poor as to neatness, accuracy, or completeness.*   Reports usually neat, accurate, and complete.*   Reports always neat, accurate, and complete.*

* Underline which. Add any related word that expresses your opinion better than the descriptive words listed here.

K. Consider the student's awareness of underlying scientific principles as exhibited in her practice.

Unaware of reasons for nursing care.	Gives some evidence of understanding principles involved.	Exhibits unusual ability in applying principles in her practice, psychological, physiological, bacteriological.*

L. Consider the administrative ability of the student. (Senior students only.)

Either makes poor plans or cannot execute them.	Moderately efficient in normal situations.	Displays outstanding administrative ability. Carries responsibility well.

II. Personal Fitness

A. Consider vitality of the student.

Appears tired and listless.	Fairly vigorous.	Extremely vigorous.

B. Consider the neatness of the student.

Untidy in personal grooming.	Usually neat.	Always neat and well groomed.

C. Consider the student's mental attitude.

Self-centered, pessimistic, rigid, critical, indifferent, aggressive.*	Generally wholesome.	Always natural and wholesome in attitude.

Indicate special handicaps and outstanding abilities not otherwise recorded. State instances indicating possession or absence of any noteworthy traits.

Signatures of:
Supervisor
Head Nurse
Student

The University of Minnesota Press
Minneapolis

Copyright, 1931, by the University of Minnesota. Price, $6.00 a thousand, plus postage.

INDEX

NOTES

16. Turn rubber sheet back upon mattress, unwashed side of rubber sheet out.
17. Clean foot of bed and springs.
18. Place rubber sheet on springs, unwashed side out.
19. Wash rest of rubber sheet.
20. Hang over top of bed.
21. Clean rest of furniture.
22. Remove cleaning materials to service room.
    a. Scour basin.
    b. Wash whisk broom in soapy solution.
    c. Clean tray and leave articles in order.
23. Wash hands.
24. Air unit 6 hours if possible.
25. Take fresh linen, including towels, to bedside.
26. Make up as closed bed.
27. Leave unit or room complete and ready for new patient.

References
Kelley, *Textbook of Nursing Technique*, p. 21.

Removal of Stains

Blood
1. Fresh blood:
   a. Soak in cold water.
   b. Wash in soap and water.
   c. Apply hydrogen peroxide.
2. Old blood:
   a. Keep wet with hydrogen peroxide and ammonia for several hours.
3. Thick blood on bedticking:
   a. Apply a thick paste of starch and water and allow to stand for several hours in the sun. Apply fresh paste when this becomes discolored. (On blankets use same treatment, but wash with Ivory soap and water.)

Ink
1. When fresh, wash out in clear water.
2. Apply dilute oxalic acid, ¼ teaspoonful to 1 cup of water. Wash out with water and repeat if necessary.
3. Alternate potassium permanganate (1 gram to 1 liter of water) and oxalic acid.
4. Soak or boil in sour milk.
5. Soak in sweet milk.
6. Apply lemon juice and salt and keep in the sun.
7. Try ammonia and alcohol.
8. Ink on carpet: apply dry salt and renew when stained.

Care of plumbing
1. Do not throw coffee grounds, hair, thread, pieces of soap, tongue blades, cotton applicators, cotton balls, sanitary pads, toothpick applicators, gauze, nor anything else that will not dissolve into hoppers, sinks, tubs, toilets, etc.
2. Report defects to head nurse at once.
3. Never allow water to run or drip from faucets; it results in an unnecessary waste of the water supply and unnecessary wear of the faucet.
4. Sodium carbonate (12 drams to 1 qt. of water) may be used in waste pipes every few days to keep them free from accumulations of grease.

Cleaning a Unit or Room after Discharge of Patient

Purpose
1. Cleanliness.
2. To remove all suggestions of preceding patient.
3. To have unit or room ready for new patient.

Necessary articles

Gray basin with hot water.	Newspaper or rubber square.
Cleaning cloths.	Whisk broom.
Mild scouring powder.	Hamper bag.
Mild soap.	Tray.

Procedure
1. Remove refuse and all unnecessary articles.
2. Bring in hamper bag.
3. Remove the linen, including towels, and place it directly into hamper.
4. Hang blankets over back of chair to air, or place them in hamper if necessary. (Consult head nurse as to care of blankets.)
5. Hang rubber sheet over foot of bed.
6. Remove hamper bag.
7. Carry articles on tray to bedside.
8. Clean upper side of mattress with dampened whisk broom. Be sure to get into all crevices.
9. Turn mattress back.
10. Clean half of under side of mattress.
11. Clean upper half of bed and springs.
12. Turn mattress back on clean half of springs.
13. Clean half of pillows with dampened whisk broom and place with clean side on mattress; then clean other side, brushing toward foot of bed.
14. Place rubber sheet on unwashed springs.
15. Wash rubber sheet and dry.

    c. Scour, wash with soap and water, rinse and dry, and place on rack.
7. Faucets:
    a. Nickel: clean with soap and water and polish.
    b. Brass: clean with metal polish.
8. Hoppers:
    a. Flush.
    b. Clean with stiff, long-handled brush.
    c. Complete cleaning with cloth, soap, and water.
    d. Remove stains.
9. Hampers:
    a. Wash thoroughly.
    b. See that bag is clean and that soiled linen is not hanging over the side.
10. Hopper brushes and bedpan mops:
    a. Wash brushes and mops under running water after use.
    b. Place brush and mop in pail of soapy solution.
    c. Clean pails thoroughly every day and refill with fresh soapy solution.
11. Sterilizer, basin and instrument:
    a. Clean inside and outside of sterilizer daily.
    b. Once a week clean by boiling; use 1 cup of sodium carbonate to ¾ sterilizer of water.
    c. Remove all loose sediment; it clogs the waste pipes.
    d. Polish outside of sterilizer daily.

References
Harmer, *Principles and Practice of Nursing*, pp. 39–45.

Care of the Bathroom and Lavatory

Purpose
1. Cleanliness and order.

Necessary articles
Cleaning cloths.
Mild soap.
Mild scouring powder.

Procedure
1. Remove soiled towels, unnecessary articles, and refuse.
2. Clean porcelain tub and washbowls with scouring powder, followed by hot water and soap.
3. Flush toilet and clean with hopper brush. Clean bowl inside and outside.
4. Clean furniture and all utensils, etc., that are left in the bathroom.

5. Arrange furniture in proper position.
6. Carry all cleaning articles to service room.
7. Wash cleaning cloths with soap and water and hang to dry in the place provided for them.
8. Leave other articles clean and in proper place.

Care of the Service Room

Purpose
1. Cleanliness and order.

Necessary articles

Gray basin with hot water.   Mild soap.
Cleaning cloths.   Mild scouring powder.

General instructions
1. Pick up and put away all articles out of place.
2. Pay attention to ventilation.

Procedure
1. Tables and utensil rack, etc.:
   a. Remove refuse and all unnecessary articles.
   b. Wash shelves and tables, etc., daily.
   c. Wipe off all bottles.
   d. Place empty drug bottles in drug basket.
2. Mouthwash cups:
   a. Rinse in service room with cold water.
   b. Boil for 10 minutes in kitchen, either in dishpan or dish sterilizer.
   c. Scour, wash with soap and water, rinse, and dry.
   d. Return to place provided for them.
3. Basins and foot tubs:
   a. Wash with cold water and place upside down in sterilizer.
   b. Boil 10 minutes.
   c. Remove from sterilizer, scour, wash with soap and water, rinse and dry.
   d. Replace on shelf.
4. Pitchers, trays, vases:
   a. Wash thoroughly after use.
   b. Dry and replace on shelf.
   c. Boil for 10 minutes when contaminated.
5. Irrigating cans:
   a. Wash thoroughly.
   b. Boil 10 minutes.
   c. Dry and replace on shelf.
6. Bedpans and urinals:
   a. Wash thoroughly with bedpan mop.
   b. Boil 10 minutes.

    d. Flush all toilets and hoppers when necessary and keep them in perfect order.

    e. Dispose of soiled dressings as soon as taken from patient.

    f. Change the water on flowers daily.

References

    Harmer, *Principles and Practice of Nursing* (3d edition, 1934), pp. 31–40.

    Kelley, *Textbook of Nursing Technique*, pp. 19–21.

    Broadhurst, *Home and Community Hygiene*, pp. 115–47.

Dusting and Cleaning

Purpose

    1. Cleanliness and order.

General instructions

    1. Have the right attitude toward the work. Cleanliness is essential to patients' recovery and nurses must not only supervise the cleaning but show a willingness to participate when necessary. A real understanding of cleaning is best obtained by doing it.

    2. Develop a system of work conserving time and energy.

    3. Be economical in care and use of materials.

    4. Clean thoroughly every day after sweeping.

    5. Clean with a firm, even, straight stroke, not round and round.

    6. Use a clean cloth and plenty of clean water and change water frequently.

    7. Do not use a wet cloth on electric fixtures and polished furniture.

    8. Furniture should be moved from painted walls before cleaning.

    9. Clean thoroughly, especially in the corners.

Necessary articles

Gray basin with water.	Mild scouring powder.
Cleaning cloths.	Newspaper or rubber square.
Mild soap.	Tray.

Procedure

    1. Fill basin half full of hot water and carry it with the other articles on a tray to room or ward.

    2. Spread the newspaper or rubber on bedside table (if necessary to protect the table) and place the articles so that they will be convenient for use.

    3. Clean the bed, tables, chairs, and dresser. Pay particular attention to springs and rungs on beds and chairs and do not forget the bars that are out of sight.

    4. Straighten articles on bedside table.

I. CLEANLINESS AND ORDER

Care and Hygiene of the Ward

Purpose
1. Cleanliness as a precaution against contamination.
2. Order as an aid to more efficient work.
3. Comfort and attractiveness.
4. Care of furniture and equipment as an aid to economy.

General instructions
1. Always have a definite plan of procedure before beginning work in a ward.
2. Keep rooms or wards well lighted, but do not leave artificial lights on if they are not needed.
3. Prevent unnecessary noise.
4. While in room always attend to immediate needs of patient.

Room or ward order
1. See that room or ward is clean and in perfect order.
   a. Adjust window shades to uniform height.
   b. Remove all refuse and place in paper bag or newspaper.
   c. Keep bedside tables free of unnecessary articles.
   d. Leave beds and chairs straight, wheels of beds turned in, towels neatly folded, stands in order with no accumulation of articles.
   e. Leave no articles on window sills, radiators, or floor.
   f. Keep beds in perfect alignment and away from the walls.
   g. When leaving the room or ward, take with you articles no longer needed.
   h. Place straight bedside chair with seat under and at foot of bed on the same side as the table.

Room or ward hygiene
1. Keep room or ward well ventilated without allowing patient to be in a draft.
   a. General ward, 68° F.
   b. Bathroom, 72° F.
   c. Surgical department, 75°–80° F.
2. Inform yourself in each hospital concerning food brought in to patients.
3. Prevent unpleasant odors.
   a. Keep bed utensils clean.
   b. Cover bedpans and urinals as soon as removed from patient and carry immediately to service room.
   c. Keep all patients and their bedding clean.

ELEMENTARY PROCEDURES

ADVANCED PROCEDURES

TABLE OF CONTENTS

ELEMENTARY PROCEDURES

ing are of widely different types and have a joint capacity of 1,292 beds. Because of the varied and complete services they offer, we believe that this manual of the procedures now being used in them will be found adapted to the use of other schools of nursing, connected with hospitals of various kinds. The hospitals associated in the school are:

1. The Minneapolis General Hospital, with 525 beds, for the care of the indigent sick of the city.
2. The Elliot Memorial, Christian and Todd Memorial, and Eustis Building — units of the University Hospital, with 400 beds, for the care of the indigent sick of the state, the treatment of patients suffering with cancer, Student Health Service, and out-patient clinics.
3. The Charles T. Miller Hospital, St. Paul, with 200 beds, for the care of private patients.
4. The Northern Pacific Beneficial Association Hospital, St. Paul, with 167 beds, for the care of private patients.

The Glen Lake Sanitorium, with 750 beds, for the care of the tuberculosis patients of the county, is affiliated with the School of Nursing.

MARION L. VANNIER
Director, School of Nursing,
University of Minnesota

PREFACE TO THE FIRST EDITION

This manual of nursing procedures was prepared originally in mimeograph form for the use of students in the University of Minnesota School of Nursing. Soon requests for copies of the book came to us from various sources: from affiliating schools of nursing, from visitors and nurse educators, and from medical students and internes preparing for general practice.

The material, therefore, was carefully revised by a committee composed of instructors resident in the four associated hospitals of the University of Minnesota School of Nursing: Barbara A. Thompson, instructor, School of Nursing, University of Minnesota; Lana Babcock, instructor, Charles T. Miller Hospital, St. Paul; Minna Schultz, instructor, Northern Pacific Beneficial Association Hospital, St. Paul; Melda Korfhage, instructor, Minneapolis General Hospital, Minneapolis; Esther Andreason, instructor, University Hospital, Minneapolis. After further testing the manual was edited and rearranged for publication in its present form by Marion L. Vannier, director of the University of Minnesota School of Nursing.

No attempt has been made to include any of the associated material given by the instructor in lectures preceding or accompanying the demonstrations. The purpose of the manual is to assure accuracy in detail and to obviate the necessity of note-taking by the students during the presentation of the demonstrations by the instructor. Harmer's *Principles and Practice of Nursing*, second edition, is the required text used in addition to this manual.

The arrangement of the material in lessons is in accordance with the plan followed in the University School. The students are taught first those procedures related to the patient's environment, then those minor duties affecting the patient which involve little responsibility, and gradually the student is taught, and allowed to carry out, the more difficult procedures.

The course covers eighty hours, divided into fifty-two hours of Elementary Practical Nursing and twenty-eight hours of Advanced Practical Nursing. Thirteen two-hour periods are used by the instructor in presenting the lectures and demonstrations of the first part, and thirteen two-hour periods are used by the students in class practice, presenting return demonstrations for the instructor's criticism. The same arrangement is carried out with the fourteen lessons in the Advanced Procedures.

The four associated hospitals of the University School of Nurs-

special diet kitchen, gynecology, communicable diseases, and out-patient clinics; (2) The Elliot Memorial, Christian and Todd Memorial, and Eustis buildings — units of the University Hospital, with 400 beds for the indigent sick of the state, offering the above services with the exception of communicable diseases and in addition the treatment of patients suffering with cancer; (3) The Charles T. Miller Hospital, St. Paul, with 200 beds for the care of private patients in medicine, surgery, and obstetrics; (4) The Glen Lake Sanatorium, with 750 beds for the care of the tuberculous patients of the county, affiliated with the School of Nursing.

In January, 1934, through the financial assistance of a C. W. A. project, and through the interest and help of Dr. Malcolm McLean, director of the General College, University of Minnesota, and Mr. Robert Kissack, head of the Department of Visual Education, moving pictures were made of certain procedures, as has been indicated in footnotes. The demonstrations were done by Miss Louise Waagen, Miss Marian Chladek serving as the patient.

Inasmuch as these pictures have been used for only one class, it is too early to comment on the success of them in the teaching of the subject.

BARBARA A. THOMPSON

PREFACE TO THE SECOND EDITION

This book has been revised after four years of use. The aim has been to describe the procedures more clearly and to list the steps in each procedure in the order that they are to be carried out by the student.

We have also omitted the following procedures, which obviously belong in a ward manual and which, by virtue of the fact that hospitals differ in their set-up, cannot be utilized in all hospitals: admission and discharge of patients, care of clothing and valuables, care and collection of specimens in detail, day and night reports, duties of the night nurse, pre-operative and post-operative care in detail, and blood transfusion. These procedures have been omitted because of the lack of uniformity in the associated hospitals. They are, however, to be prepared in the same form as the other procedures, mimeographed, and distributed to the students when the procedures are taught.

The hours of formal class work devoted to the course in Principles and Practice of Nursing are 140. Of these, 99 are class and 41 are laboratory hours. This course includes lettering, bandaging, hospital economy, and massage.

Among the faculty of the University of Minnesota School of Nursing to whom we are especially indebted are Miss Florence Parisa, instructor in the General Hospital; Miss Cecelia Hauge, instructor in the University Hospital; Miss Elizabeth Sands, formerly instructor in the Charles T. Miller Hospital; Miss Louise Waagen, present instructor in the Charles T. Miller Hospital; and Miss Ida MacDonald, assistant instructor in the General Hospital. For the procedures on communicable disease technique we are grateful to Miss Ruth Johnson, teaching supervisor in the Communicable Disease Department of the General Hospital. Others of the faculty who have made helpful suggestions and criticisms are: Miss Katharine J. Densford, director; Miss Lucile Petry, assistant professor; and Mrs. Dorothy Kurtzman, formerly superintendent of nurses, University Hospital; and the teaching supervisors and head nurses in all the associated hospitals. In addition, we are especially appreciative of the helpfulness of Mrs. Mary Marvin Wayland.

Since the publication of the last edition the Northern Pacific Beneficial Association Hospital has discontinued taking students. The set-up, therefore, is as follows: (1) The Minneapolis General Hospital, with 650 beds for the care of the indigent sick of the city, offering medicine, surgery, obstetrics, pediatrics, operating room,

A Textbook of
Nursing Technique

A MANUAL USED IN THE ASSOCIATED HOSPITALS IN THE UNIVERSITY OF MINNESOTA SCHOOL OF NURSING

MARION L. VANNIER, R.N.

FORMERLY SUPERINTENDENT OF NURSES, UNIVERSITY HOSPITAL, AND DIRECTOR OF THE SCHOOL OF NURSING, UNIVERSITY OF MINNESOTA

BARBARA A. THOMPSON, R.N., B.S.

DIRECTOR OF THE WISCONSIN BUREAU OF NURSING EDUCATION
FORMERLY ASSISTANT SUPERINTENDENT OF NURSES, UNIVERSITY HOSPITAL, MINNEAPOLIS,
TEACHING SUPERVISOR OF SURGICAL NURSING, PRESBYTERIAN HOSPITAL, CHICAGO, AND
SUPERINTENDENT OF NURSES, GENERAL HOSPITAL, MINNEAPOLIS

Second Edition Revised

1935

THE UNIVERSITY OF MINNESOTA PRESS
MINNEAPOLIS

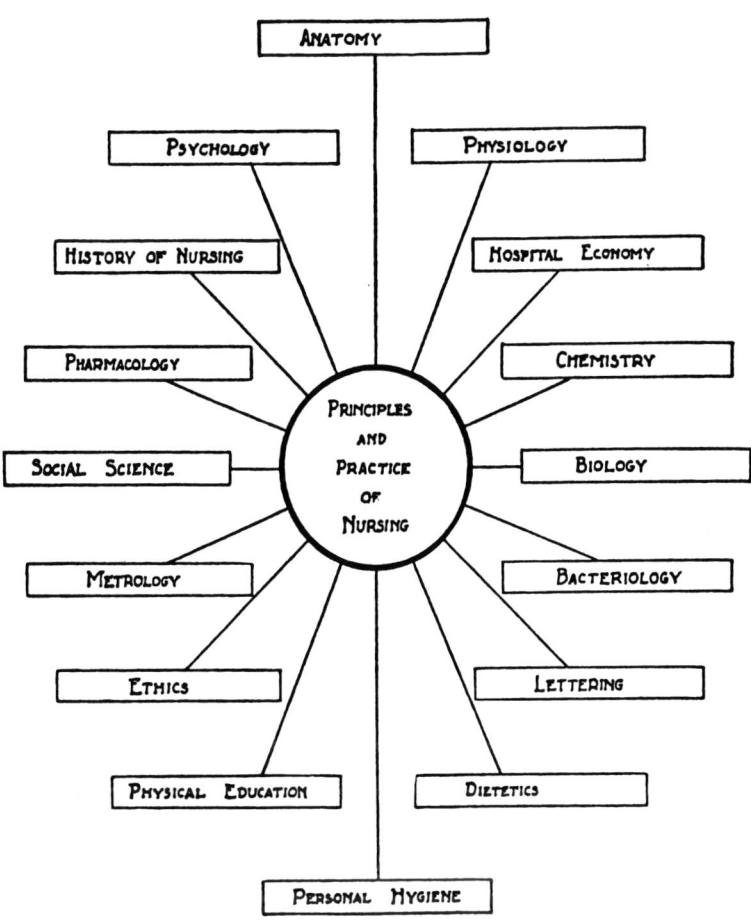

ANATOMY

PSYCHOLOGY   PHYSIOLOGY

HISTORY OF NURSING   HOSPITAL ECONOMY

PHARMACOLOGY   CHEMISTRY

SOCIAL SCIENCE   PRINCIPLES AND PRACTICE OF NURSING   BIOLOGY

METROLOGY   BACTERIOLOGY

ETHICS   LETTERING

PHYSICAL EDUCATION   DIETETICS

PERSONAL HYGIENE

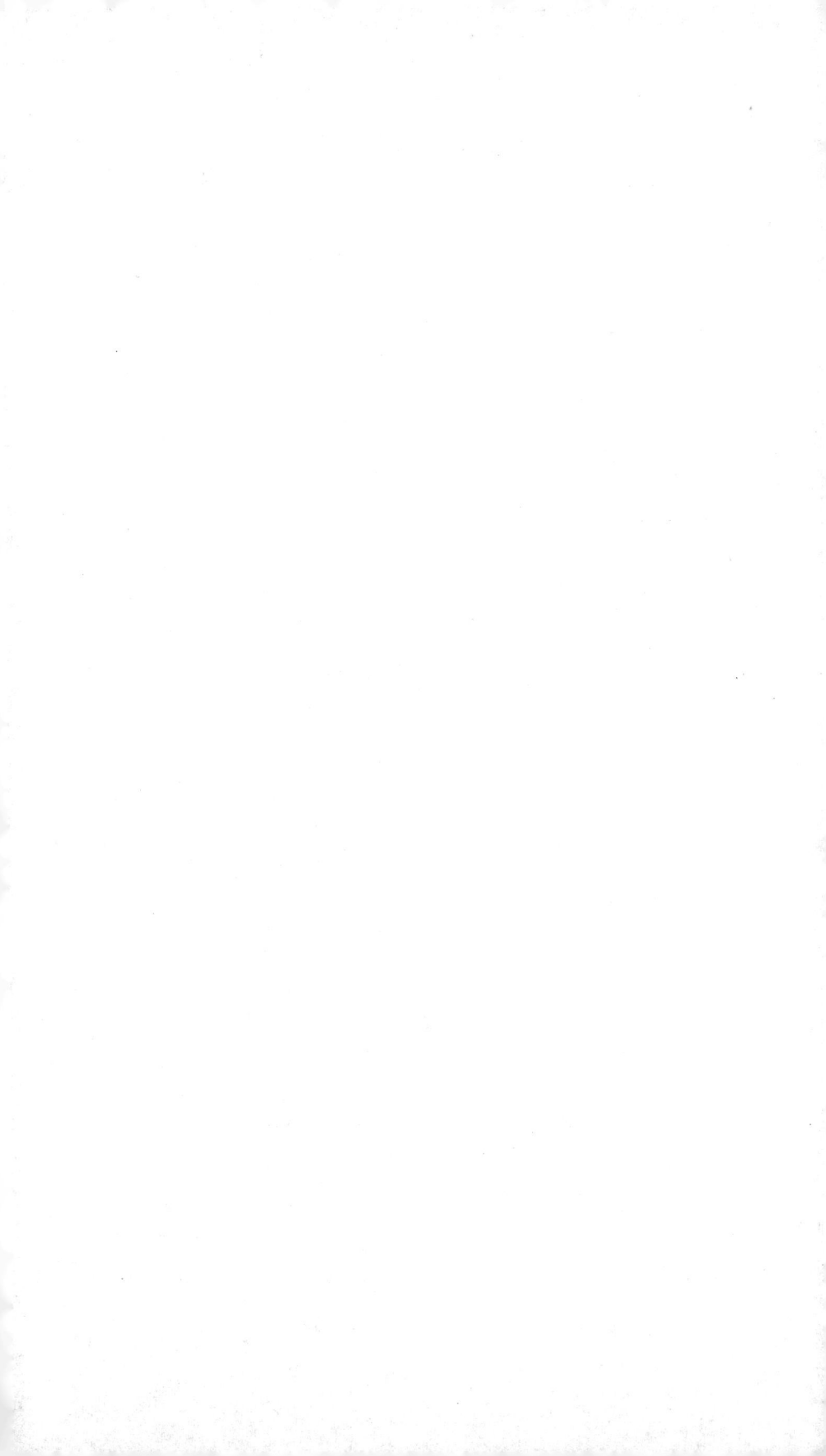